WATCH YOUR
WEIGHT COOKBOOK

Healthy and Delicious Recipes for Rapid Weight Loss. Including Point Value, Full Color Image, Health Benefit, and Meal Plan.

Dr. Taylah Waller

Copyright © 2024 Taylah Waller

Disclaimer:

The recipes and information provided in this cookbook are for general informational purposes only. While every effort has been made to ensure the accuracy and completeness of the material, the author and publisher make no representations or warranties of any kind, explicit or implied, regarding the appropriateness, reliability, or availability of the recipes or information included herein for any purpose.

It is recommended that readers exercise their discretion and judgment while creating and consuming foods based on the recipes presented in this handbook. The author and publisher will not be responsible for any loss, injury, or damage resulting from the use of this cookbook or the recipes included within.

Please be aware that certain recipes may include common allergens such as nuts, dairy, eggs, gluten, and others. The reader must check the ingredients and take appropriate measures if they have allergies or dietary restrictions.

Consultation with a certified healthcare expert is suggested before making any substantial changes to your diet or lifestyle based on the information presented in this cookbook.

Contents

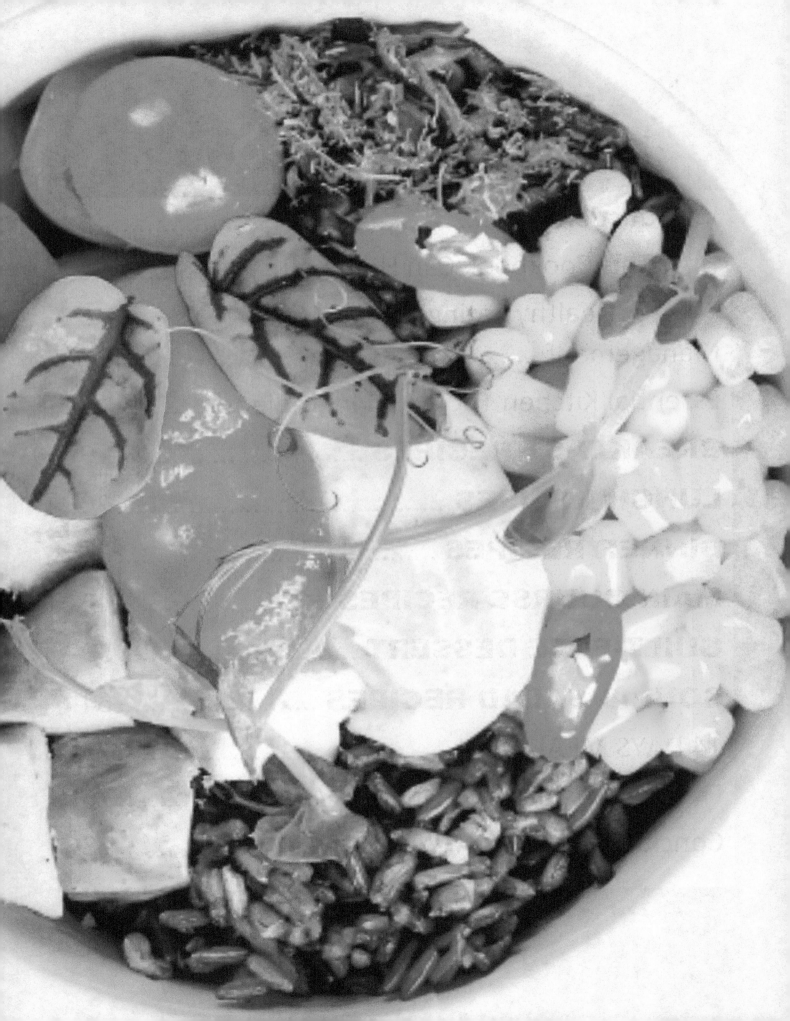

Introduction

Welcome to the "WATCH YOUR WEIGHT COOKBOOK," where tasty cuisine and mindful eating collide. We set out on a path to a healthier you, one recipe at a time, in these pages. I know how difficult it can be to manage weight healthily and still keep a balanced diet because I work as a nutritionist. This cookbook is more than simply a list of recipes; it's a resource created to give you wholesome choices that support your health objectives.

Each recipe in this cookbook is meticulously crafted with your health in mind. Whether you're starting your day with a nourishing breakfast, enjoying a satisfying lunch, or savoring a guilt-free dessert, every dish comes with a clear understanding of its nutritional impact. You'll find that every recipe is accompanied by point values, ensuring you can make informed choices that support your journey towards a healthier lifestyle.

Healthy eating shouldn't mean sacrificing flavor or enjoyment. That's why the recipes in this book are as delicious as they are nutritious. From vibrant salads to hearty main courses and tempting desserts, each dish is a testament to the idea that eating well can be both satisfying and beneficial. By making small, sustainable changes to your diet, you can discover a renewed sense of energy, confidence, and well-being.

In addition to our collection of recipes, you'll find practical tips and guidance on meal planning, essential ingredients for your kitchen, and substitutions to tailor recipes to your preferences and dietary needs. This cookbook is more than just a compilation of meals—it's a resource designed to support you on your path to a healthier lifestyle.

As you embark on this culinary adventure with me, remember that every recipe here is a step towards a healthier, more balanced life. Whether you're cooking for yourself, your family, or friends, these dishes are crafted to nourish both body and soul. So, let's embrace the joy of cooking and eating well together. Here's to good food, good health, and a journey towards a happier, healthier you.

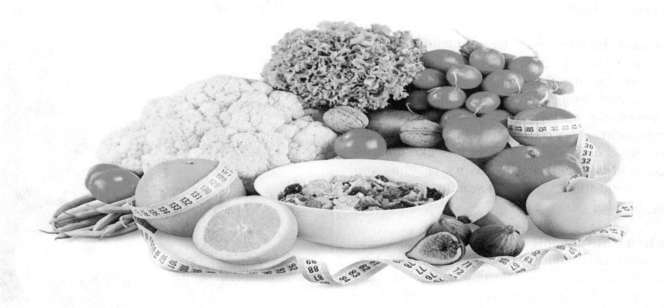

How This Cookbook Can Help You

In navigating the journey toward weight management, this cookbook serves as your dedicated companion, offering a meticulously curated collection of recipes and practical guidance designed to support your goals effectively.

Nutritional Balance and Point Values: Each recipe presented here is not only delicious but also nutritionally balanced. By providing point values for each recipe, you are empowered to make informed choices that align with your weight management objectives. Whether you are seeking a hearty breakfast, a fulfilling lunch, a flavorful dinner, or a guilt-free dessert, the recipes in this cookbook are crafted to nourish your body while supporting your efforts in managing weight.

Emphasis on Holistic Health: Beyond mere caloric considerations, this cookbook places a significant emphasis on your overall health and well-being. The recipes feature wholesome ingredients that are rich in essential nutrients, fiber, and vitamins. These elements are crucial in promoting satiety, enhancing your energy levels throughout the day, and facilitating your pursuit of a balanced lifestyle.

Practical Insights and Recommendations: In addition to the recipes, you will find practical guidance on meal planning, essential kitchen staples, and thoughtful substitutions tailored to accommodate various dietary preferences and requirements. This cookbook equips you with the necessary knowledge and tools to make mindful choices in your culinary endeavors, enabling you to create nutritious meals that seamlessly integrate into your daily routine.

Fostering Sustainable Habits: Sustainable weight management is a journey that emphasizes enduring lifestyle changes over fleeting solutions. The strategies and recipes featured in this cookbook are thoughtfully curated to support you in establishing and maintaining healthy eating habits. By embracing a diverse array of wholesome and satisfying meals, you will cultivate a positive relationship with food while advancing towards your weight management aspirations in a sustainable and gratifying manner.

Building a Supportive Community: Recognizing that wellness is a collective endeavor, this cookbook is part of a community dedicated to health and vitality. Whether you are preparing meals for yourself, your loved ones, or your friends, the recipes within these pages are intended to be shared and enjoyed together. They serve as a catalyst for forging meaningful connections and reaffirming your commitment to a healthier lifestyle.

In embracing the resources and insights presented in this cookbook, you are embarking on a transformative journey towards enhanced well-being and vitality. It is my sincere hope that these recipes and recommendations will empower you to navigate your weight management goals with confidence, resilience, and joy.

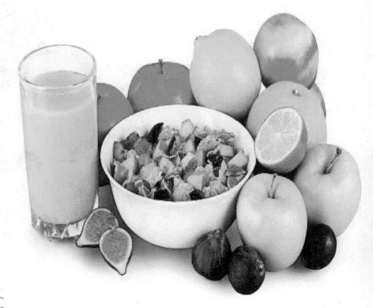

Tips for Healthy Eating and Weight Management

Achieving and maintaining a healthy weight involves more than just counting calories—it's about adopting sustainable habits that promote overall well-being. Here are some practical tips to support you on your journey:

Eat Mindfully: Pay attention to your body's hunger and fullness cues. Avoid distractions while eating, such as watching TV or scrolling through your phone, to fully enjoy and savor your meals.

Focus on Whole Foods: Incorporate plenty of fruits, vegetables, whole grains, lean proteins, and healthy fats into your diet. These nutrient-dense foods provide essential vitamins, minerals, and fiber to support optimal health.

Watch Portion Sizes: Be mindful of portion sizes to avoid overeating. Use smaller plates and bowls, and take your time to enjoy each bite. This helps prevent consuming more calories than your body needs.

Stay Hydrated: Drink plenty of water throughout the day. Sometimes thirst can be mistaken for hunger, so staying hydrated can help curb unnecessary snacking.

Plan and Prepare Meals: Take time to plan your meals and snacks for the week ahead. This allows you to make healthier choices and avoid impulse eating. Batch cooking and preparing meals in advance can also save time and promote healthier eating habits.

Limit Processed Foods and Sugary Drinks: Reduce your intake of processed foods high in added sugars, unhealthy fats, and sodium. Opt for whole, unprocessed foods whenever possible and choose water or herbal tea over sugary drinks.

Be Active: Incorporate regular physical activity into your routine. Aim for at least 150 minutes of moderate-intensity exercise per week, such as brisk walking, swimming, or cycling. Physical activity not only supports weight management but also promotes overall health and well-being.

Practice Self-Care: Manage stress and emotions without turning to food. Practice relaxation techniques such as deep breathing, yoga, or meditation to help reduce stress levels and promote a balanced mindset.

Seek Support: Surround yourself with a supportive network of friends, family, or professionals who can encourage and motivate you on your journey. Sharing your goals and progress with others can help keep you accountable and motivated.

Celebrate Progress: Focus on making gradual, sustainable changes rather than aiming for perfection. Celebrate your successes, no matter how small, and acknowledge the positive steps you are taking towards a healthier lifestyle.

By incorporating these tips into your daily routine, you can cultivate healthier eating habits and achieve your weight management goals in a way that is enjoyable and sustainable.

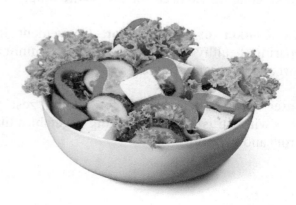

Essential Kitchen Tools

Chef's Knife: A high-quality chef's knife makes chopping fruits, vegetables, and proteins easier and safer.

Cutting Boards: Have separate cutting boards for meat, poultry, fish, and vegetables to prevent cross-contamination.

Measuring Cups and Spoons: Accurate measuring tools ensure portion control and consistent cooking results.

Non-Stick Skillet or Pan: Ideal for cooking with minimal oil or butter, making it easier to prepare healthy meals.

Steamer Basket: Great for steaming vegetables while preserving their nutrients and natural flavors.

Baking Sheets and Ovenware: Essential for roasting vegetables, baking lean proteins, and preparing healthy snacks.

Blender or Food Processor: Perfect for creating smoothies, soups, sauces, and homemade dips with fresh ingredients.

Salad Spinner: Ensures crisp and dry greens for salads, reducing the need for excess dressing.

Slow Cooker or Instant Pot: Convenient for preparing healthy one-pot meals with minimal effort and maximum flavor.

Grater and Zester: Useful for adding zest to dishes with citrus fruits and grating vegetables like carrots and zucchini.

Essential Ingredients

Whole Grains: Brown rice, quinoa, oats, whole wheat pasta—provide fiber and sustained energy.

Lean Proteins: Skinless poultry, lean cuts of beef or pork, tofu, tempeh, beans, and legumes—support muscle health and satiety.

Fresh Vegetables: Leafy greens (spinach, kale), cruciferous vegetables (broccoli, cauliflower), colorful peppers, tomatoes—packed with vitamins, minerals, and antioxidants.

Fresh Fruits: Berries, apples, oranges, bananas—provide natural sweetness and essential nutrients.

Healthy Fats: Olive oil, avocado, nuts (almonds, walnuts), seeds (chia, flaxseed)—support heart health and provide satiety.

Herbs and Spices: Fresh herbs (basil, cilantro), garlic, ginger, turmeric, cumin—add flavor without extra calories or sodium.

Low-Sodium Broth or Stock: Use as a base for soups, stews, and sauces to enhance flavor without added salt.

Greek Yogurt and Low-Fat Dairy: Substitute for sour cream or heavy cream in recipes for added protein and creaminess.

Natural Sweeteners: Honey, maple syrup, stevia—use sparingly to sweeten dishes and beverages.

Healthy Snacks: Air-popped popcorn, rice cakes, raw nuts, and seeds—provide nutrient-rich options between meals.

1

BREAKFAST RECIPES

For good reason, breakfast is frequently cited as the most significant meal of the day. It speeds up your metabolism, gives your body the nutrition it needs, and establishes a positive example for making better decisions all day long. With the aid of our scrumptious and nourishing breakfast recipes from this cookbook, you may begin your day full of vitality and enthusiasm.

Every breakfast recipe is designed to help you reach your weight loss objectives by providing well-balanced, high-protein, high-fiber, and healthy-fat meals. Together, these nutrients help you feel full and satisfied throughout the day, which lessens the chance that you'll seek junk food later on. You may effortlessly monitor your consumption and make well-informed decisions that comply with your diet plan by using the point values provided for every recipe.

Our breakfast department offers a wide range of meals to suit all tastes and preferences, from satisfying whole grain alternatives to refreshing smoothies and robust egg white scrambles loaded with veggies. These recipes will support you in adopting a healthier lifestyle from the first meal, whether you have a slow morning or need a quick, on-the-go option. Take some time to explore these delicious and nutritious breakfast recipes that can help you on your weight management path and give you energy in the mornings.

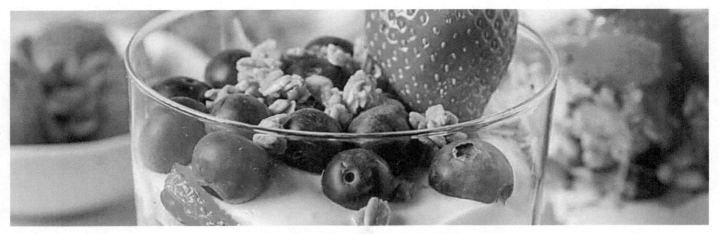

Greek Yogurt Parfait with Fresh Berries

COOKING TIME: 0 MIN | PREP TIME: 5 MIN | TOTAL TIME: 5 MIN | SERVING SIZE: 1

INGREDIENTS:

- 1/2 cup non-fat Greek yogurt
- 1/2 cup fresh mixed berries (such as strawberries, blueberries, raspberries)
- 1 tablespoon honey
- 2 tablespoons granola
- Fresh mint leaves for garnish

INSTRUCTIONS:

1. Prepare the Yogurt: In a serving glass or bowl, spoon half of the Greek yogurt.
2. Add Berries: Layer half of the fresh mixed berries on top of the yogurt.
3. Repeat Layers: Repeat with the remaining Greek yogurt and fresh berries.
4. Top with Granola: Sprinkle granola evenly over the top layer of berries.
5. Garnish (optional): Garnish with fresh mint leaves for added freshness and presentation.
6. Serve: Enjoy immediately as a nutritious and satisfying breakfast option.

Nutritional Information (per serving):

Calories: 250 kcal

Protein: 18g

Carbohydrates: 40g

Fat: 3g

Fiber: 6g

Sugar: 26g

HEALTH BENEFITS:

Greek yogurt is high in protein, which helps keep you full and supports muscle repair. Fresh berries are rich in antioxidants, vitamins, and fiber, which aid in digestion and boost your immune system. This parfait is a balanced breakfast that promotes gut health and sustained energy levels.

POINT VALUE:

4

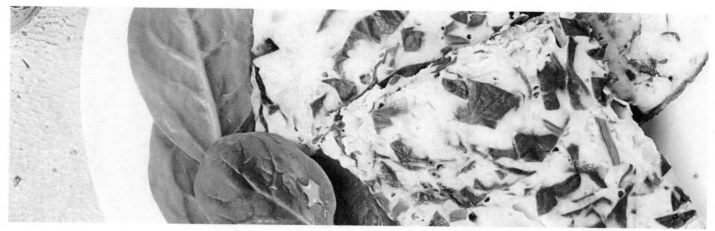

Spinach and Mushroom Egg White Omelette

COOKING TIME: 10 MIN | PREP TIME: 5 MIN | TOTAL TIME: 15 MIN | SERVING SIZE: 1

INGREDIENTS:

- 1 cup egg whites (about 6 egg whites)
- 1 cup fresh spinach leaves, chopped
- 1/2 cup sliced mushrooms
- 1/4 cup diced onions
- 1 garlic clove, minced
- Salt and pepper, to taste
- Cooking spray or 1 teaspoon olive oil

INSTRUCTIONS:

1. Preparation: In a medium bowl, whisk together the egg whites until frothy. Season with a pinch of salt and pepper. Set aside.
2. Chop the spinach leaves, slice the mushrooms, dice the onions, and mince the garlic clove.
3. Cooking: Heat a non-stick skillet over medium heat and lightly coat with cooking spray or olive oil.
4. Add the diced onions to the skillet and sauté for 2-3 minutes until they begin to soften.
5. Add the sliced mushrooms to the skillet and cook for another 2-3 minutes until they are tender and lightly browned.
6. Add the minced garlic and chopped spinach to the skillet. Cook for 1-2 minutes until the spinach wilts.
7. Omelette Assembly: Pour the whisked egg whites evenly over the vegetables in the skillet.
8. Allow the omelette to cook undisturbed for 3-4 minutes, or until the edges start to set.
9. Folding: Using a spatula, gently lift the edges of the omelette and tilt the skillet to let any uncooked egg whites flow to the edges.
10. Final Touch: Once the omelette is mostly set with a slightly runny center, carefully fold it in half using the spatula.
11. Cook for another 1-2 minutes, or until the omelette is fully cooked through and no longer runny.
12. Serving: Slide the omelette onto a plate and serve immediately, garnished with a sprinkle of fresh herbs if desired.

HEALTH BENEFITS:

Egg whites are an excellent source of lean protein without the added cholesterol found in yolks. Spinach is packed with iron, vitamins A and C, and antioxidants, while mushrooms provide important nutrients such as selenium and vitamin D. This omelette supports muscle health, boosts immunity, and aids in weight management.

POINT VALUE:

3

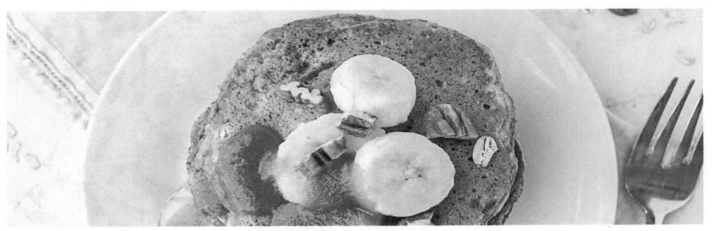

Whole Grain Pancakes with Banana and Walnuts

COOKING TIME: 15 MIN | PREP TIME: 10 MIN | TOTAL TIME: 25 MIN | SERVING SIZE: 2

INGREDIENTS:

- 1/2 cup whole wheat flour
- 1/4 cup rolled oats
- 1 teaspoon baking powder
- Pinch of salt
- 1/2 cup unsweetened almond milk (or milk of choice)
- 1 tablespoon maple syrup
- 1/2 teaspoon vanilla extract
- 1 ripe banana, mashed
- 1/4 cup chopped walnuts
- Cooking spray or oil for the pan

INSTRUCTIONS:

1. In a large mixing bowl, combine the whole wheat flour, rolled oats, baking powder, and salt.
2. In a separate bowl, whisk together the almond milk, maple syrup, and vanilla extract.
3. Pour the wet ingredients into the dry ingredients and stir until just combined. Fold in the mashed banana and chopped walnuts.
4. Heat a non-stick skillet or griddle over medium heat. Lightly coat with cooking spray or a small amount of oil.
5. Pour about 1/4 cup of batter onto the skillet for each pancake. Cook until bubbles form on the surface and the edges look set, about 2-3 minutes.
6. Carefully flip the pancakes and cook for another 1-2 minutes, or until golden brown and cooked through.
7. Serve warm, topped with additional sliced banana, a sprinkle of walnuts, and a drizzle of maple syrup if desired.

HEALTH BENEFITS:

Whole grains provide sustained energy and are rich in fiber, promoting digestive health. Bananas offer potassium and natural sweetness without added sugars. Walnuts are a good source of healthy fats, omega-3 fatty acids, and antioxidants, which support heart health and brain function.

POINT VALUE:

5

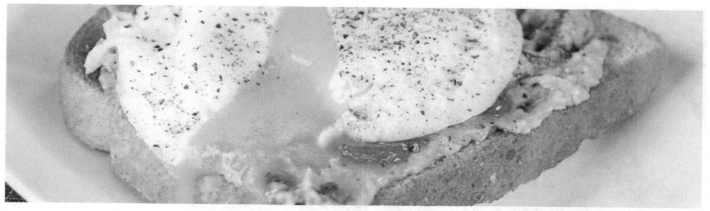

Avocado Toast with Poached Egg

COOKING TIME: 10 MIN | PREP TIME: 5 MIN | TOTAL TIME: 15 MIN | SERVING SIZE: 1

INGREDIENTS:

- 1 slice whole grain bread (60 grams)
- 1/2 ripe avocado
- 1 large egg
- Salt and pepper to taste
- Optional: Red pepper flakes or hot sauce for added spice (not included in point calculation)

INSTRUCTIONS:

1. Prepare the Avocado: Slice the avocado in half, remove the pit, and scoop the flesh into a small bowl. Mash the avocado with a fork until smooth. Season with salt and pepper to taste.
2. Toast the Bread: Toast the slice of whole grain bread until golden and crispy.
3. Poach the Egg: Fill a small saucepan with water and bring it to a gentle simmer over medium heat. Crack the egg into a small bowl.
4. Carefully slide the egg into the simmering water. Poach the egg for about 3-4 minutes, until the white is set but the yolk is still runny.
5. Remove the egg with a slotted spoon and drain excess water on a paper towel.
6. Assemble the Avocado Toast: Spread the mashed avocado evenly onto the toasted bread slice.
7. Add the Poached Egg: Carefully place the poached egg on top of the mashed avocado.
8. Season and Serve: Season the poached egg with a pinch of salt and pepper. Optionally, garnish with red pepper flakes or hot sauce for added flavor.

HEALTH BENEFITS:

Avocados are rich in healthy monounsaturated fats, which are good for heart health. They also provide fiber, potassium, and vitamins. Poached eggs add high-quality protein and essential amino acids, making this a nutrient-dense breakfast that promotes satiety and balanced blood sugar levels.

POINT VALUE:

4

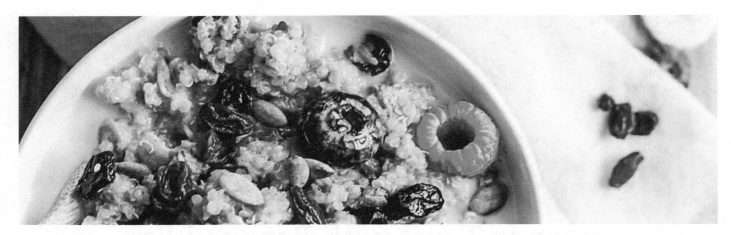

Quinoa Breakfast Bowl with Almond Butter and Fruit

COOKING TIME: 20 MIN | PREP TIME: 10 MIN | TOTAL TIME: 30 MIN | SERVING SIZE: 1

INGREDIENTS:

- 1/2 cup cooked quinoa
- 1 tablespoon almond butter
- 1/2 banana, sliced
- 1/2 cup mixed berries (such as strawberries, blueberries, raspberries)
- 1 tablespoon chopped almonds
- 1 teaspoon honey (optional, not included in points)

INSTRUCTIONS:

1. Prepare Quinoa: Cook quinoa according to package instructions. Allow it to cool slightly before assembling the breakfast bowl.
2. Assemble Breakfast Bowl: In a serving bowl, add cooked quinoa as the base.
3. Add Toppings: Spread almond butter over the quinoa. Arrange sliced banana and mixed berries on top.
4. Finish with Almonds: Sprinkle chopped almonds over the fruit.
5. Optional Sweetener: Drizzle with honey if desired for added sweetness (not included in points).
6. Serve: Enjoy your nutritious and satisfying quinoa breakfast bowl immediately.

HEALTH BENEFITS:

Quinoa is a complete protein, providing all nine essential amino acids, and is high in fiber and magnesium. Almond butter adds healthy fats, protein, and vitamin E. Fresh fruit provides vitamins, antioxidants, and natural sugars for a balanced and energizing breakfast.

POINT VALUE:

6

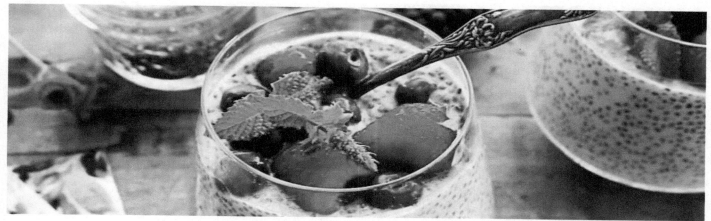

Chia Seed Pudding with Berries

COOKING TIME: 0 MIN | PREP TIME: 5 MIN | TOTAL TIME: 4 HRS | SERVING SIZE: 1

INGREDIENTS:

- 2 tablespoons chia seeds
- 1/2 cup unsweetened almond milk (or any milk of your choice)
- 1/2 teaspoon vanilla extract
- 1 teaspoon honey or maple syrup (optional, adjust to taste)
- 1/2 cup mixed berries (such as strawberries, blueberries, raspberries)

INSTRUCTIONS:

1. In a mixing bowl, combine chia seeds, almond milk, vanilla extract, and honey or maple syrup (if using). Stir well to combine.
2. Cover the bowl and refrigerate for at least 4 hours or overnight, stirring once or twice during the first hour to prevent clumping.
3. After chilling, the chia seeds will have absorbed the liquid and the mixture will have a pudding-like consistency.
4. To serve, layer the chia seed pudding with mixed berries in a serving glass or bowl.
5. Enjoy immediately as a nutritious and satisfying breakfast option.

HEALTH BENEFITS:

Chia seeds are a powerhouse of omega-3 fatty acids, fiber, and protein. They also help in maintaining hydration and promote heart health. Berries add a rich source of antioxidants and vitamins, making this pudding an excellent choice for a nutrient-dense and satisfying meal.

POINT VALUE:

3

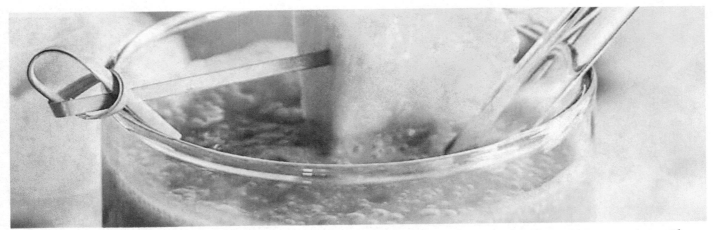

Green Smoothie with Spinach and Pineapple

COOKING TIME: 0 MIN | PREP TIME: 5 MIN | TOTAL TIME: 5 MIN | SERVING SIZE: 1

INGREDIENTS:

- 1 cup fresh spinach leaves
- 1/2 cup frozen pineapple chunks
- 1/2 medium banana
- 1/2 cup unsweetened almond milk
- 1 tablespoon chia seeds
- 1 teaspoon honey (optional, not included in point value)

INSTRUCTIONS:

1. Prepare Ingredients: Wash the spinach leaves thoroughly. Peel and slice the banana into chunks if not already done. Measure out the almond milk and chia seeds.
2. Blend Ingredients: In a blender, combine the fresh spinach leaves, frozen pineapple chunks, banana, almond milk, and chia seeds.
3. Blend until Smooth: Blend on high speed until the mixture is smooth and creamy, ensuring all ingredients are well combined.
4. Adjust Consistency (if needed): If the smoothie is too thick, add a little more almond milk. If it's too thin, add a few more pineapple chunks or banana pieces.
5. Serve Immediately: Pour the green smoothie into a glass and enjoy immediately for maximum freshness and flavor.

Nutritional Information (per serving):

Calories: 220 kcal

Protein: 5g

Carbohydrates: 40g

Fiber: 8g

Sugars: 21g

Fat: 6g

Saturated Fat: 1g

HEALTH BENEFITS:

Spinach is rich in iron, calcium, and vitamins A and C, which support overall health and immunity. Pineapple provides vitamin C, manganese, and digestive enzymes. This green smoothie is refreshing, hydrating, and helps detoxify the body while boosting energy levels.

POINT VALUE:

4

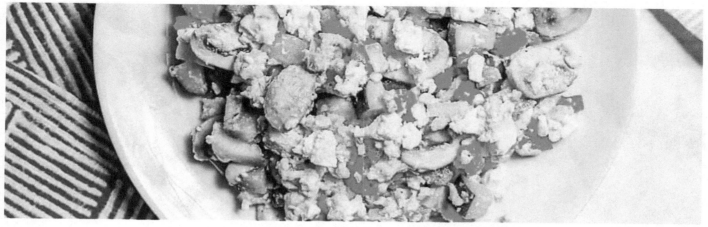

Veggie Egg White Scramble

COOKING TIME: 10 MIN | PREP TIME: 5 MIN | TOTAL TIME: 15 MIN | SERVING SIZE: 1

INGREDIENTS:

- 1 cup egg whites
- 1/2 cup diced bell peppers (any color)
- 1/4 cup diced onions
- 1/4 cup diced tomatoes
- 1/4 cup baby spinach leaves
- Salt and pepper to taste
- Cooking spray or olive oil spray

INSTRUCTIONS:

1. Heat a non-stick skillet over medium heat and lightly coat with cooking spray or olive oil spray.
2. Add diced bell peppers and onions to the skillet. Sauté for 2-3 minutes until they begin to soften.
3. Stir in diced tomatoes and baby spinach leaves. Cook for another 1-2 minutes until spinach is wilted.
4. Pour egg whites over the vegetables in the skillet. Season with salt and pepper to taste.
5. Cook, stirring occasionally, until the egg whites are fully cooked and scrambled, about 4-5 minutes.
6. Remove from heat and transfer the Veggie Egg White Scramble to a serving plate.
7. Serve hot, garnished with fresh herbs if desired. Enjoy your nutritious and satisfying breakfast!

HEALTH BENEFITS:

Egg whites provide lean protein essential for muscle maintenance and repair. The mixed vegetables add fiber, vitamins, and antioxidants, promoting digestive health and boosting the immune system. This scramble is a low-calorie, nutrient-rich breakfast option.

POINT VALUE:

3

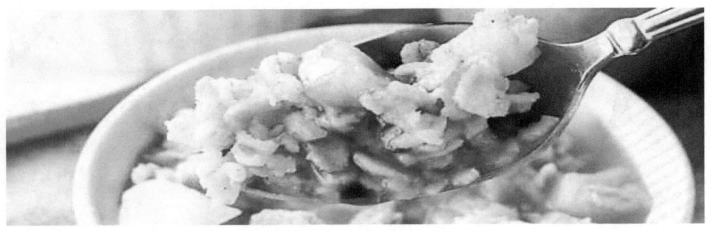

Oatmeal with Apples and Cinnamon

COOKING TIME: 15 MIN | PREP TIME: 5 MIN | TOTAL TIME: 20 MIN | SERVING SIZE: 1

INGREDIENTS:

- 1/2 cup rolled oats
- 1 cup water
- 1/2 cup unsweetened almond milk
- 1 medium apple, peeled, cored, and chopped
- 1/2 teaspoon ground cinnamon
- 1 teaspoon honey (optional, not included in point value)
- Pinch of salt

INSTRUCTIONS:

1. In a small saucepan, bring water to a boil.
2. Stir in rolled oats and reduce heat to low. Simmer for 5 minutes, stirring occasionally.
3. Add almond milk, chopped apple, cinnamon, and a pinch of salt to the oats. Cook for an additional 5-7 minutes, or until the oats are creamy and the apples are tender.
4. Remove from heat and let sit for 1-2 minutes to thicken.
5. Transfer oatmeal to a bowl. Drizzle with honey if desired (not included in point value).
6. Serve warm and enjoy your comforting bowl of oatmeal with apples and cinnamon!

HEALTH BENEFITS:

Oatmeal is high in soluble fiber, which helps reduce cholesterol levels and promotes heart health. Apples provide vitamins, fiber, and antioxidants, while cinnamon has anti-inflammatory properties and helps regulate blood sugar levels. This combination makes for a heart-healthy and satisfying breakfast.

POINT VALUE:

4

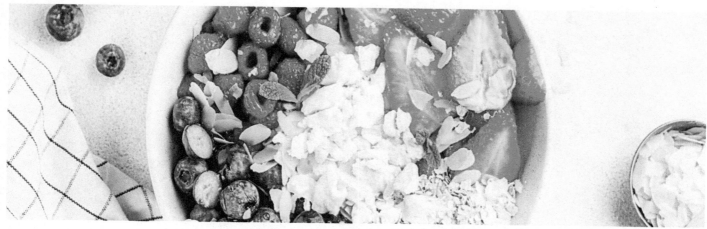

Cottage Cheese and Fruit Bowl

COOKING TIME: 0 MIN | PREP TIME: 5 MIN | TOTAL TIME: 5 MIN | SERVING SIZE: 1

INGREDIENTS:

- 1/2 cup low-fat cottage cheese
- 1/2 cup fresh mixed berries (such as strawberries, blueberries, raspberries)
- 1/4 cup diced fresh pineapple
- 1 tablespoon sliced almonds
- 1 teaspoon honey (optional, not included in points)

INSTRUCTIONS:

1. In a breakfast bowl, scoop out 1/2 cup of low-fat cottage cheese.
2. Wash and prepare 1/2 cup of fresh mixed berries. Add the berries to the bowl with the cottage cheese.
3. Dice 1/4 cup of fresh pineapple into small pieces and add them to the bowl.
4. Sprinkle 1 tablespoon of sliced almonds over the top of the cottage cheese and fruit.
5. Drizzle 1 teaspoon of honey over the bowl if desired (note: honey is optional and not included in the point value).
6. Enjoy your nutritious and delicious Cottage Cheese and Fruit Bowl!

Nutritional Information (per serving):

Calories: Approximately 210 kcal
Protein: 15g
Carbohydrates: 25g
Fiber: 4g

HEALTH BENEFITS:

Cottage cheese is high in protein and calcium, supporting bone health and muscle maintenance. Fresh fruit adds vitamins, fiber, and antioxidants, aiding in digestion and boosting the immune system. This bowl is a balanced, low-calorie option that keeps you full and energized.

POINT VALUE:

3

2

LUNCH RECIPES

Lunchtime offers a crucial opportunity to refuel your body and sustain your energy levels throughout the day. In this section, you'll discover a diverse array of lunch recipes designed specifically to support your weight loss journey. Each recipe is crafted with wholesome ingredients that are rich in nutrients and flavor, ensuring that your midday meal is both satisfying and nourishing.

Our lunch recipes emphasize balance and variety, incorporating lean proteins, whole grains, fresh vegetables, and healthy fats. Whether you're looking for a light and refreshing salad, a hearty soup, or a flavorful wrap, these recipes will help you stay on track with your weight management goals without sacrificing taste or enjoyment. With clear point values provided for each dish, you'll have the tools you need to make mindful choices and enjoy a fulfilling lunch that aligns with your health objectives.

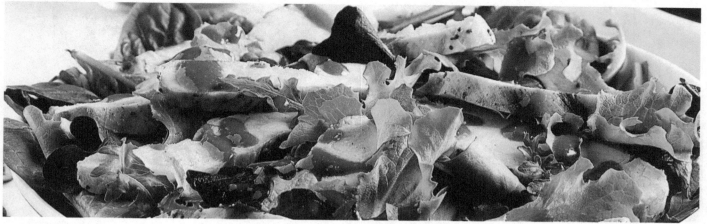

Grilled Chicken Salad with Balsamic Vinaigrette

COOKING TIME: 15 MIN | PREP TIME: 10 MIN | TOTAL TIME: 25 MIN | SERVING SIZE: 1

INGREDIENTS:

- 4 oz boneless, skinless chicken breast
- Salt and pepper, to taste
- 2 cups mixed salad greens (such as spinach, arugula, and romaine)
- 1/2 cup cherry tomatoes, halved
- 1/4 cup cucumber, sliced
- 1/4 cup red onion, thinly sliced
- 1 tablespoon balsamic vinegar
- 1 teaspoon Dijon mustard
- 1 teaspoon honey (optional, not included in points)
- 1 tablespoon extra-virgin olive oil

INSTRUCTIONS:

1. Preheat grill or grill pan over medium-high heat.
2. Season the chicken breast with salt and pepper.
3. Grill the chicken breast for about 6-7 minutes per side, or until fully cooked and no longer pink in the center. Remove from heat and let it rest for a few minutes before slicing.
4. In a large salad bowl, combine the mixed salad greens, cherry tomatoes, cucumber, and red onion slices.
5. In a small bowl, whisk together balsamic vinegar, Dijon mustard, and olive oil until well combined to make the vinaigrette.
6. Slice the grilled chicken breast into thin slices.
7. Arrange the sliced chicken breast on top of the salad greens.
8. Drizzle the balsamic vinaigrette over the salad and toss gently to coat.
9. Serve immediately and enjoy your flavorful and satisfying Grilled Chicken Salad!

Nutritional Information (per serving):

Calories: Approximately 300 kcal

Protein: 30g

Carbohydrates: 4g

Fiber: 1g

Sugars: 1g

HEALTH BENEFITS:

Grilled chicken is a lean source of protein, which helps in muscle maintenance and repair. The mixed greens and vegetables in the salad provide essential vitamins, minerals, and fiber, supporting digestive health and satiety. Balsamic vinaigrette adds flavor with minimal calories.

POINT VALUE:

5

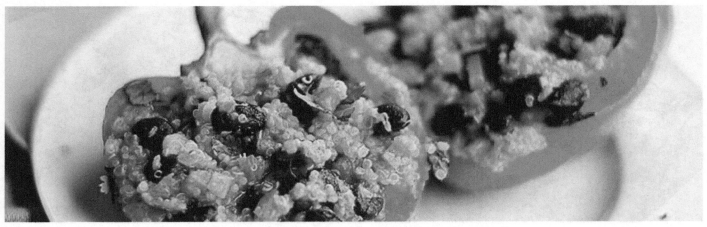

Quinoa Stuffed Bell Peppers

COOKING TIME: 40 MIN | PREP TIME: 20 MIN | TOTAL TIME: 1 HRS | SERVING SIZE: 4

INGREDIENTS:

- 4 large bell peppers (any color)
- 1 cup quinoa, rinsed
- 2 cups vegetable broth
- 1 tablespoon olive oil
- 1 onion, finely chopped
- 2 cloves garlic, minced
- 1 can (15 ounces) black beans, drained and rinsed
- 1 can (15 ounces) diced tomatoes, drained
- 1 teaspoon ground cumin
- 1 teaspoon chili powder
- Salt and pepper, to taste
- 1/2 cup shredded cheddar cheese (optional, not included in points)

INSTRUCTIONS:

1. Preheat your oven to 375°F (190°C). Grease a baking dish large enough to fit all 4 bell peppers.
2. Cut the tops off the bell peppers and remove the seeds and membranes. Place the peppers upright in the prepared baking dish.
3. In a medium saucepan, bring the vegetable broth to a boil. Add the quinoa, reduce the heat to low, cover, and simmer for about 15 minutes or until the quinoa is cooked and the broth is absorbed.
4. In a large skillet, heat the olive oil over medium heat. Add the chopped onion and sauté until softened, about 5 minutes. Add the minced garlic and cook for another 1-2 minutes until fragrant.
5. Stir in the black beans, diced tomatoes, ground cumin, and chili powder. Season with salt and pepper to taste. Cook for another 5 minutes, allowing the flavors to meld together.
6. Remove the skillet from the heat and stir in the cooked quinoa until well combined.
7. Spoon the quinoa mixture evenly into the hollowed-out bell peppers, pressing gently to pack the filling.
8. Cover the baking dish with foil and bake in the preheated oven for 25-30 minutes, or until the bell peppers are tender.
9. Optional: Remove the foil, sprinkle shredded cheddar cheese on top of each stuffed pepper, and return to the oven for another 5 minutes or until the cheese is melted and bubbly (note: cheese is optional and not included in the point value).
10. Remove from the oven and let cool slightly before serving.

HEALTH BENEFITS:

Quinoa is a complete protein, rich in fiber and essential amino acids. Bell peppers are loaded with vitamins A and C, antioxidants, and fiber. This dish is filling and nutritious, promoting overall health and supporting weight loss goals.

POINT VALUE:

6

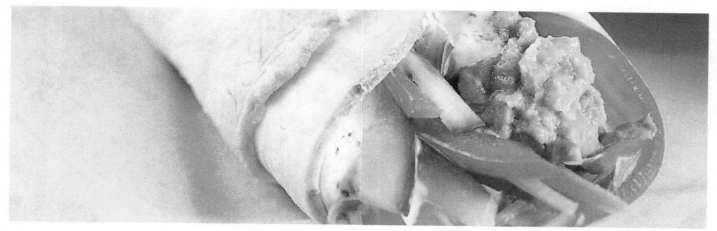

Turkey and Avocado Wrap

COOKING TIME: 0 MIN | PREP TIME: 10 MIN | TOTAL TIME: 10 MIN | SERVING SIZE: 1

INGREDIENTS:

- 1 whole wheat tortilla (8 inches in diameter)
- 2 ounces sliced deli turkey breast
- 1/4 avocado, thinly sliced
- 1/4 cup shredded lettuce
- 2 slices tomato
- 1 tablespoon hummus
- Salt and pepper to taste

INSTRUCTIONS:

1. Lay the whole wheat tortilla flat on a clean surface.
2. Spread 1 tablespoon of hummus evenly over the tortilla, leaving a small border around the edges.
3. Layer the sliced deli turkey breast evenly over the hummus.
4. Arrange the thinly sliced avocado, shredded lettuce, and tomato slices on top of the turkey.
5. Season with salt and pepper to taste.
6. Fold in the sides of the tortilla, then roll it up tightly from bottom to top to create a wrap.
7. Slice the wrap in half diagonally if desired, and serve immediately.

Nutritional Information (per wrap):
Calories: Approximately 280 kcal

Protein: 20g

Carbohydrates: 26g

Fiber: 7g

HEALTH BENEFITS:
Turkey is a lean protein that helps in muscle growth and repair, while avocado provides healthy fats, fiber, and a variety of vitamins and minerals. This wrap is a balanced, satisfying meal that keeps you full and energized.

POINT VALUE:

4

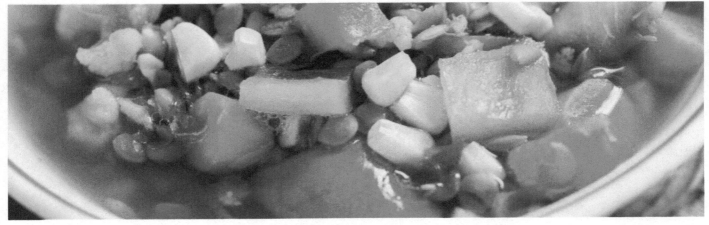

Lentil and Vegetable Soup

COOKING TIME: 30 MIN | PREP TIME: 15 MIN | TOTAL TIME: 45 MIN | SERVING SIZE: 4

INGREDIENTS:

- 1 cup dried green or brown lentils, rinsed and drained
- 1 tablespoon olive oil
- 1 onion, diced
- 2 carrots, diced
- 2 celery stalks, diced
- 2 cloves garlic, minced
- 1 teaspoon ground cumin
- 1/2 teaspoon ground turmeric
- 1/2 teaspoon paprika
- 1/4 teaspoon cayenne pepper (optional, adjust to taste)
- 4 cups low-sodium vegetable broth
- 2 cups water
- 1 (14.5 oz) can diced tomatoes (no salt added)
- Salt and pepper, to taste
- Fresh parsley or cilantro, chopped (for garnish)

INSTRUCTIONS:

1. Heat olive oil in a large pot over medium heat. Add diced onion, carrots, and celery. Cook, stirring occasionally, until vegetables are softened, about 5-7 minutes.
2. Add minced garlic, ground cumin, turmeric, paprika, and cayenne pepper (if using). Cook for another 1-2 minutes until fragrant.
3. Add rinsed lentils, vegetable broth, water, and diced tomatoes (including juices) to the pot. Bring to a boil, then reduce heat to low and simmer, covered, for 25-30 minutes or until lentils and vegetables are tender.
4. Season with salt and pepper to taste. If the soup is too thick, you can add more water or broth to reach your desired consistency.
5. Serve hot, garnished with fresh parsley or cilantro if desired.

Nutritional Information (per serving):

Calories: Approximately 250 kcal

Protein: 14g

Carbohydrates: 40g

Fiber: 16g

HEALTH BENEFITS:

Lentils are high in protein, fiber, and essential nutrients like iron and folate. The vegetables add a variety of vitamins and minerals, making this soup nutrient-dense and low in calories. It's a hearty and healthy option for weight management.

POINT VALUE:

3

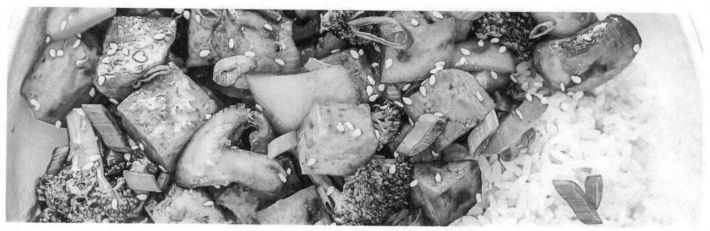

Asian-Inspired Tofu Stir-Fry

COOKING TIME: 15 MIN | PREP TIME: 15 MIN | TOTAL TIME: 30 MIN | SERVING SIZE: 1

INGREDIENTS:

- 1/2 block (about 200g) extra-firm tofu, drained and cubed
- 1 cup mixed vegetables (such as bell peppers, broccoli, snap peas)
- 1/2 cup cooked brown rice
- 1 tablespoon low-sodium soy sauce
- 1 teaspoon sesame oil
- 1 teaspoon grated fresh ginger
- 1 clove garlic, minced
- 1/2 tablespoon cornstarch mixed with 1 tablespoon water (for thickening)
- Fresh cilantro or green onions for garnish (optional, not included in points)

INSTRUCTIONS:

1. Prepare the Tofu: Press the tofu to remove excess water. Cut the tofu into cubes.
2. Cook the Tofu: Heat a non-stick skillet over medium heat. Add the tofu cubes and cook until golden and crispy on all sides, about 8-10 minutes. Remove tofu from the skillet and set aside.
3. Prepare the Vegetables: In the same skillet, add a bit of water or vegetable broth (about 2 tablespoons) and stir-fry the mixed vegetables until tender-crisp, about 5 minutes.
4. Combine Ingredients: Return the tofu to the skillet with the vegetables. Add soy sauce, sesame oil, grated ginger, and minced garlic. Stir to combine.
5. Thicken the Sauce: Pour the cornstarch mixture into the skillet and stir well. Cook for another 1-2 minutes until the sauce thickens and coats the tofu and vegetables evenly.
6. Serve: Serve the Asian-Inspired Tofu Stir-Fry over cooked brown rice.
7. Garnish (optional): Garnish with fresh cilantro or green onions if desired (note: garnishes are optional and not included in the point value).

Nutritional Information (per serving):

Calories: Approximately 380 kcal

Protein: 20g

Carbohydrates: 45g

Fiber: 7g

HEALTH BENEFITS:

Tofu is a plant-based protein that contains all essential amino acids. The mixed vegetables in the stir-fry provide a range of vitamins, minerals, and antioxidants. This dish is low in calories but high in nutrients, supporting overall health and weight loss.

POINT VALUE:

5

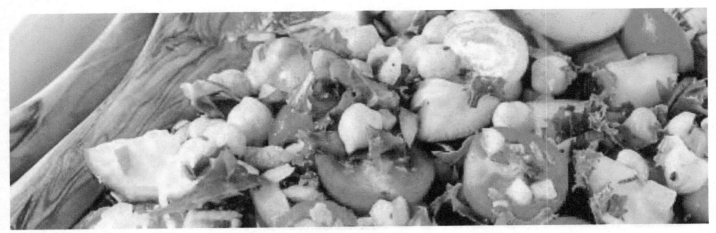

Chickpea Salad with Lemon Tahini Dressing

COOKING TIME: 0 MIN | PREP TIME: 15 MIN | TOTAL TIME: 15 MIN | SERVING SIZE: 1

INGREDIENTS:

- 1 cup canned chickpeas, drained and rinsed
- 1/2 cucumber, diced
- 1/2 red bell pepper, diced
- 1/4 cup cherry tomatoes, halved
- 2 tablespoons finely chopped red onion
- 2 tablespoons chopped fresh parsley
- 1 tablespoon tahini
- Juice of 1/2 lemon
- 1 tablespoon olive oil
- Salt and pepper to taste

INSTRUCTIONS:

1. In a large mixing bowl, combine the drained and rinsed chickpeas, diced cucumber, diced red bell pepper, cherry tomatoes, red onion, and fresh parsley.
2. In a small bowl, whisk together the tahini, lemon juice, and olive oil until smooth and creamy.
3. Pour the tahini dressing over the chickpea salad and toss gently to coat all the ingredients evenly.
4. Season with salt and pepper to taste.
5. Transfer the salad to a serving plate or bowl.
6. Enjoy your nutritious and flavorful Chickpea Salad with Lemon Tahini Dressing!

Nutritional Information (per serving):

Calories: Approximately 380 kcal

Protein: 14g

Carbohydrates: 42g

Fiber: 12g

HEALTH BENEFITS:

Chickpeas are a great source of plant-based protein and fiber, aiding in digestion and satiety. The lemon tahini dressing adds healthy fats and a burst of flavor, making this salad both nutritious and satisfying.

POINT VALUE:

4

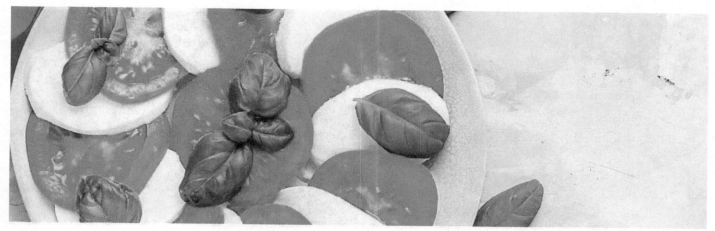

Caprese Salad with Balsamic Glaze

COOKING TIME: 0 MIN | PREP TIME: 10 MIN | TOTAL TIME: 10 MIN | SERVING SIZE: 1

INGREDIENTS:

- 1 large tomato, sliced
- 4-6 fresh basil leaves
- 2 oz fresh mozzarella cheese, sliced
- 1 teaspoon extra virgin olive oil
- 1 teaspoon balsamic glaze
- Salt and pepper to taste

INSTRUCTIONS:

1. Arrange the sliced tomatoes and fresh mozzarella cheese alternately on a serving plate.
2. Tuck fresh basil leaves between the tomato and mozzarella slices.
3. Drizzle 1 teaspoon of extra virgin olive oil evenly over the salad.
4. Drizzle 1 teaspoon of balsamic glaze over the salad.
5. Season with salt and pepper to taste.
6. Serve immediately and enjoy your light and flavorful Caprese Salad!

Nutritional Information (per serving):
Calories: Approximately 180 kcal
Protein: 10g
Carbohydrates: 7g
Fiber: 1g

HEALTH BENEFITS:
Fresh tomatoes and mozzarella provide vitamins C and K, calcium, and protein. Basil adds antioxidants, and the balsamic glaze offers a touch of sweetness with minimal calories. This light salad is refreshing and beneficial for weight management.

POINT VALUE:

3

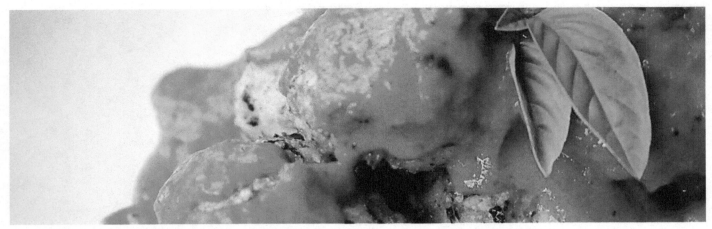

Turkey and Spinach Meatballs in Marinara Sauce

COOKING TIME: 25 MIN | PREP TIME: 15 MIN | TOTAL TIME: 40 MIN | SERVING SIZE: 4

INGREDIENTS:

- 1 lb lean ground turkey
- 1 cup fresh spinach, finely chopped
- 1/4 cup whole wheat breadcrumbs
- 1/4 cup grated Parmesan cheese
- 1 egg
- 1 teaspoon dried oregano
- 1/2 teaspoon garlic powder
- Salt and pepper to taste
- 2 cups marinara sauce (store-bought or homemade)

INSTRUCTIONS:

1. Preheat your oven to 400°F (200°C). Lightly grease a baking sheet with cooking spray or olive oil.
2. In a large mixing bowl, combine the lean ground turkey, finely chopped fresh spinach, whole wheat breadcrumbs, grated Parmesan cheese, egg, dried oregano, garlic powder, salt, and pepper.
3. Use your hands to gently mix all ingredients until well combined, being careful not to over mix.
4. Shape the mixture into approximately 16 meatballs, each about 1.5 inches in diameter, and place them on the prepared baking sheet.
5. Bake the meatballs in the preheated oven for 15-20 minutes, or until cooked through and lightly browned.
6. While the meatballs are baking, heat the marinara sauce in a large skillet over medium heat.
7. Once the meatballs are cooked, transfer them to the skillet with the marinara sauce. Gently stir to coat the meatballs with the sauce.
8. Allow the meatballs to simmer in the marinara sauce for 5-10 minutes, stirring occasionally, until heated through.
9. Serve the Turkey and Spinach Meatballs in Marinara Sauce hot, garnished with additional grated Parmesan cheese if desired.

Nutritional Information (per serving):
Calories: Approximately 300 kcal
Protein: 28g
Carbohydrates: 14g
Fiber: 3g

HEALTH BENEFITS:

Turkey is a lean protein that supports muscle health. Spinach is rich in iron, vitamins, and antioxidants. The marinara sauce adds lycopene and other nutrients from tomatoes. This dish is hearty and nutritious, promoting satiety and health.

POINT VALUE:

5

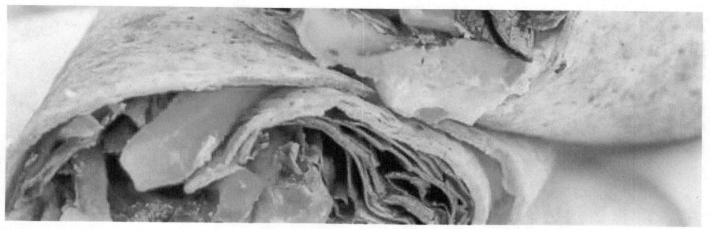

Mediterranean Veggie Wrap with Hummus

COOKING TIME: 0 MIN | PREP TIME: 10 MIN | TOTAL TIME: 10 MIN | SERVING SIZE: 1

INGREDIENTS:

- 1 large whole wheat or spinach tortilla (about 8 inches in diameter)
- 2 tablespoons hummus (store-bought or homemade)
- 1/2 cup mixed greens (such as spinach or arugula)
- 1/4 cup sliced cucumber
- 1/4 cup diced tomatoes
- 1/4 cup sliced red bell pepper
- 2 tablespoons crumbled feta cheese
- 1 tablespoon sliced Kalamata olives

INSTRUCTIONS:

1. Lay the tortilla flat on a clean surface.
2. Spread 2 tablespoons of hummus evenly over the entire surface of the tortilla.
3. Layer 1/2 cup of mixed greens, 1/4 cup sliced cucumber, 1/4 cup diced tomatoes, and 1/4 cup sliced red bell pepper on top of the hummus.
4. Sprinkle 2 tablespoons of crumbled feta cheese and 1 tablespoon of sliced Kalamata olives over the vegetables.
5. Fold the sides of the tortilla inward, then roll it up tightly from the bottom to form a wrap.
6. Slice the wrap in half diagonally, if desired, and serve immediately.

Nutritional Information (per wrap):
Calories: Approximately 300 kcal
Protein: 10g
Carbohydrates: 40g
Fiber: 7g

HEALTH BENEFITS:
This wrap is packed with fiber-rich vegetables and protein from hummus. The veggies provide essential vitamins and minerals, while hummus adds healthy fats. It's a balanced and satisfying meal that supports weight loss and overall well-being.

POINT VALUE:

4

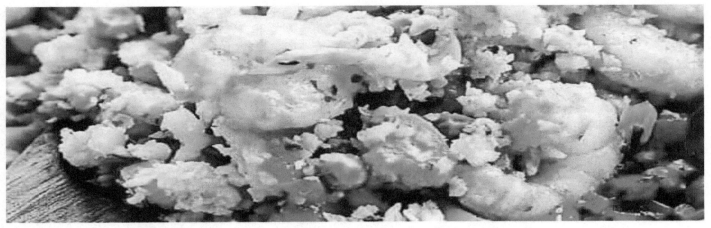

Cauliflower Fried Rice with Shrimp

COOKING TIME: 15 MIN | PREP TIME: 10 MIN | TOTAL TIME: 25 MIN | SERVING SIZE: 2

INGREDIENTS:

- 1 small head cauliflower, grated or finely chopped (about 4 cups)
- 8 oz raw shrimp, peeled and deveined
- 1 cup mixed vegetables (such as diced bell peppers, peas, carrots)
- 2 cloves garlic, minced
- 2 green onions, chopped
- 2 eggs, lightly beaten
- 2 tablespoons low-sodium soy sauce
- 1 tablespoon sesame oil
- 1 tablespoon olive oil
- Salt and pepper to taste

INSTRUCTIONS:

1. In a large skillet or wok, heat olive oil over medium-high heat. Add minced garlic and cook for 30 seconds until fragrant.
2. Add shrimp to the skillet and cook until pink and opaque, about 3-4 minutes. Remove shrimp from skillet and set aside.
3. In the same skillet, add mixed vegetables and cook for 3-4 minutes until tender-crisp.
4. Push the vegetables to one side of the skillet and pour the beaten eggs into the empty space. Scramble the eggs until cooked through, then mix with the vegetables.
5. Add grated cauliflower to the skillet, along with soy sauce and sesame oil. Stir well to combine all ingredients.
6. Cook the cauliflower fried rice for 5-6 minutes, stirring occasionally, until the cauliflower is tender and heated through.
7. Add the cooked shrimp back to the skillet and toss everything together. Season with salt and pepper to taste.
8. Divide the Cauliflower Fried Rice with Shrimp between two plates and garnish with chopped green onions.
9. Serve hot and enjoy your flavorful and satisfying lunch!

Nutritional Information (per serving):
Calories: Approximately 300 kcal
Protein: 28g
Carbohydrates: 17g
Fiber: 6g

HEALTH BENEFITS:
Cauliflower is a low-carb, low-calorie vegetable rich in vitamins and fiber. Shrimp provides lean protein and essential nutrients like selenium and iodine. This dish is a nutritious and flavorful alternative to traditional fried rice, aiding in weight loss.

POINT VALUE:

6

3

DINNER RECIPES

Each recipe in this section has been carefully crafted with a balance of lean proteins, fresh vegetables, and healthy fats to provide you with the essential nutrients your body needs. We've included point values for each recipe, making it easy for you to track your intake and stay on course with your weight management journey.

Whether you're in the mood for a hearty baked salmon, a comforting turkey and sweet potato skillet, or a light and zesty lemon garlic shrimp with zucchini noodles, you'll find a diverse range of options to suit your tastes and preferences. Our recipes are straightforward, with clear instructions to ensure you can create delicious dinners with ease.

We believe that eating healthy should be enjoyable, and these dinner recipes are here to prove that you don't have to sacrifice taste or satisfaction to achieve your weight loss goals. So, let's get cooking and transform your evenings with meals that delight your palate and nourish your body!

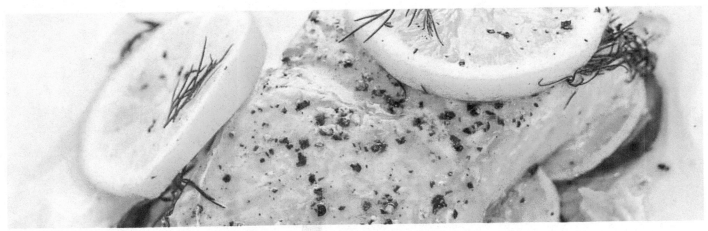

Baked Salmon with Dill and Lemon

COOKING TIME: 15 MIN | PREP TIME: 10 MIN | TOTAL TIME: 25 MIN | SERVING SIZE: 2

INGREDIENTS:

- 2 salmon fillets (about 6 oz each)
- 1 lemon, thinly sliced
- 2 tablespoons fresh dill, chopped
- 2 cloves garlic, minced
- 1 tablespoon olive oil
- Salt and pepper to taste

INSTRUCTIONS:

1. Preheat Oven: Preheat your oven to 400°F (200°C).
2. Prepare Baking Dish: Lightly grease a baking dish with a small amount of olive oil.
3. Season Salmon: Place the salmon fillets in the baking dish. Drizzle 1 tablespoon of olive oil over the fillets, and season with salt and pepper.
4. Add Garlic and Dill: Sprinkle the minced garlic evenly over the salmon fillets. Then, generously top with the chopped fresh dill.
5. Lemon Slices: Arrange the thinly sliced lemon over the top of the salmon fillets. The lemon will add a burst of citrus flavor and help keep the fish moist during baking.
6. Bake: Place the baking dish in the preheated oven and bake for 12-15 minutes, or until the salmon is cooked through and flakes easily with a fork.
7. Serve: Remove the salmon from the oven and let it rest for a minute. Serve the baked salmon fillets hot, garnished with additional fresh dill if desired

Nutritional Information (per serving):

Calories: Approximately 300 kcal

Protein: 30g

Carbohydrates: 4g

Fiber: 1g

HEALTH BENEFITS:

Salmon is rich in omega-3 fatty acids, which promote heart health and reduce inflammation. It's also a great source of high-quality protein and essential vitamins like vitamin D and B12. The dill and lemon add flavor without extra calories, making this a nutritious and delicious meal.

POINT VALUE:

6

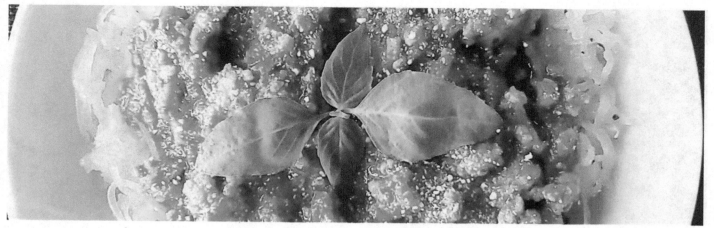

Spaghetti Squash with Turkey Bolognese

COOKING TIME: 40 MIN | PREP TIME: 15 MIN | TOTAL TIME: 55 MIN | SERVING SIZE: 4

INGREDIENTS:

- 1 large spaghetti squash
- 1 lb ground turkey (preferably lean)
- 1 can (14.5 oz) diced tomatoes, no salt added
- 1 small onion, finely chopped
- 2 cloves garlic, minced
- 1 carrot, finely diced
- 1 celery stalk, finely diced
- 1/2 cup low-sodium chicken broth
- 2 tablespoons tomato paste
- 1 teaspoon dried oregano
- 1 teaspoon dried basil
- 1/2 teaspoon salt
- 1/4 teaspoon black pepper
- 1 tablespoon olive oil
- Fresh parsley, chopped (for garnish)

HEALTH BENEFITS:

Spaghetti squash is low in calories and carbohydrates, providing a healthy alternative to traditional pasta. The lean ground turkey is a great source of protein and lower in fat compared to beef. This dish is also rich in vitamins and minerals, particularly from the tomato-based sauce.

INSTRUCTIONS:

1. Preheat your oven to 400°F (200°C). Carefully cut the spaghetti squash in half lengthwise and scoop out the seeds. Place the halves cut side down on a baking sheet lined with parchment paper. Bake for 35-40 minutes or until the squash is tender and can be easily shredded with a fork.
2. While the squash is baking, heat olive oil in a large skillet over medium heat. Add the chopped onion, carrot, and celery, and sauté for 5-7 minutes until the vegetables are softened.
3. Add the minced garlic to the skillet and cook for another 1-2 minutes until fragrant.
4. Add the ground turkey to the skillet and cook until browned, breaking it up into small pieces with a wooden spoon as it cooks.
5. Stir in the tomato paste, diced tomatoes, chicken broth, dried oregano, dried basil, salt, and black pepper. Bring the mixture to a simmer and cook for 15-20 minutes, allowing the flavors to meld together and the sauce to thicken.
6. Once the spaghetti squash is done baking, remove it from the oven and let it cool slightly. Use a fork to scrape out the strands of squash into a large bowl, creating spaghetti-like strands.
7. Divide the spaghetti squash among four plates and top each with a generous portion of turkey bolognese sauce.
8. Garnish with freshly chopped parsley for a burst of color and freshness.
9. Serve hot and enjoy your delicious, low-carb Spaghetti Squash with Turkey Bolognese!

POINT VALUE:

5

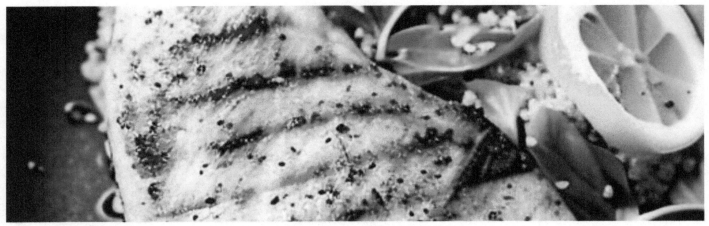

Grilled Lemon Herb Chicken with Quinoa

COOKING TIME: 20 MIN | PREP TIME: 10 MIN | TOTAL TIME: 30 MIN | SERVING SIZE: 2

INGREDIENTS:

- 2 boneless, skinless chicken breasts (about 6 oz each)
- 1 cup quinoa, uncooked
- 2 cups low-sodium chicken broth
- 1 lemon (juice and zest)
- 2 tablespoons olive oil
- 2 cloves garlic, minced
- 1 teaspoon dried oregano
- 1 teaspoon dried thyme
- 1/2 teaspoon salt
- 1/4 teaspoon black pepper
- Fresh parsley, chopped (for garnish)

INSTRUCTIONS:

1. Prepare the Marinade: In a small bowl, combine the juice and zest of one lemon, olive oil, minced garlic, dried oregano, dried thyme, salt, and black pepper. Mix well to create the marinade.
2. Marinate the Chicken: Place the chicken breasts in a shallow dish or a resealable plastic bag. Pour the marinade over the chicken, ensuring both sides are well-coated. Let it marinate for at least 10 minutes, or up to 1 hour for more flavor.
3. Cook the Quinoa: While the chicken is marinating, rinse the quinoa under cold water. In a medium saucepan, bring the low-sodium chicken broth to a boil. Add the quinoa, reduce the heat to low, cover, and simmer for 15 minutes or until the quinoa is cooked and the liquid is absorbed. Fluff with a fork and set aside.
4. Grill the Chicken: Preheat a grill or grill pan over medium-high heat. Remove the chicken from the marinade and discard any remaining marinade. Grill the chicken breasts for 6-7 minutes on each side, or until fully cooked and the internal temperature reaches 165°F (74°C). The chicken should be golden brown with a slightly charred exterior.
5. Serve: Divide the cooked quinoa between two plates. Place one grilled chicken breast on each plate. Garnish with fresh parsley for a burst of color and added freshness.
6. Enjoy: Serve the Grilled Lemon Herb Chicken with Quinoa hot. Relish the harmonious blend of flavors, the zestiness of the lemon, the aromatic herbs, and the nutty quinoa.

HEALTH BENEFITS:

Chicken is a lean protein that supports muscle maintenance and growth. Quinoa is a complete protein and rich in fiber, which aids in digestion and helps keep you full longer. The lemon and herbs provide antioxidants and enhance flavor without adding extra calories.

POINT VALUE:

6

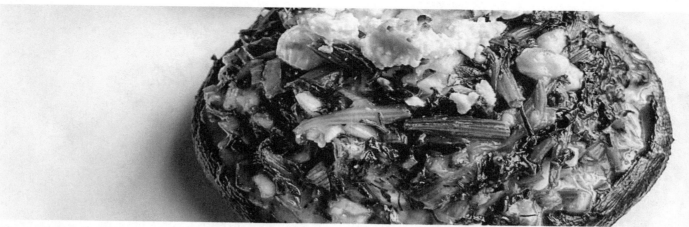

Stuffed Portobello Mushrooms with Spinach and Feta

COOKING TIME: 25 MIN | PREP TIME: 15 MIN | TOTAL TIME: 40 MIN | SERVING SIZE: 2

INGREDIENTS:

- 4 large Portobello mushrooms
- 2 cups fresh spinach, chopped
- 1/2 cup crumbled feta cheese
- 1/4 cup diced red bell pepper
- 2 cloves garlic, minced
- 2 tablespoons olive oil
- 1/2 teaspoon dried oregano
- Salt and pepper to taste

INSTRUCTIONS:

1. Preheat your oven to 400°F (200°C). Line a baking sheet with parchment paper.
2. Remove the stems from the Portobello mushrooms and gently scrape out the gills with a spoon. Place mushrooms on the prepared baking sheet, gill side up.
3. In a large skillet, heat 1 tablespoon of olive oil over medium heat. Add minced garlic and sauté for 30 seconds until fragrant.
4. Add chopped spinach and diced red bell pepper to the skillet. Cook for 3-4 minutes until spinach is wilted and peppers are tender.
5. Remove skillet from heat and stir in crumbled feta cheese, dried oregano, salt, and pepper.
6. Divide the spinach and feta mixture evenly among the Portobello mushrooms, filling each cap generously.
7. Drizzle the stuffed mushrooms with the remaining tablespoon of olive oil.
8. Bake in the preheated oven for 20-25 minutes, or until the mushrooms are tender and the filling is heated through.
9. Remove from the oven and let cool slightly before serving.
10. Enjoy your flavorful Stuffed Portobello Mushrooms with Spinach and Feta as a satisfying and nutritious dinner!

Nutritional Information (per serving): Calories: Approximately 220 kcal, Protein: 12g

Carbohydrates: 12g

Fiber: 4g

HEALTH BENEFITS:

Portobello mushrooms are low in calories and high in fiber, making them filling and nutritious. Spinach is packed with vitamins A, C, and K, as well as iron and calcium. Feta adds a savory flavor and some calcium, while keeping the overall dish light.

POINT VALUE:

4

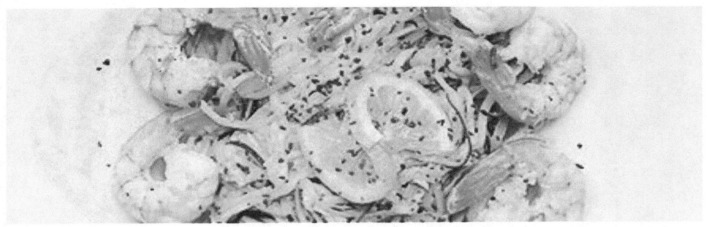

Lemon Garlic Shrimp with Zucchini Noodles

COOKING TIME: 15 MIN | PREP TIME: 10 MIN | TOTAL TIME: 25 MIN | SERVING SIZE: 2

INGREDIENTS:

- 8 oz raw shrimp, peeled and deveined
- 2 medium zucchinis
- 2 tablespoons olive oil
- 3 cloves garlic, minced
- 1/2 teaspoon red pepper flakes (optional)
- Zest and juice of 1 lemon
- Salt and pepper to taste
- Fresh parsley, chopped, for garnish

INSTRUCTIONS:

1. Using a spiralizer or vegetable peeler, create zucchini noodles (zoodles) from the zucchinis. Set aside.
2. Heat 1 tablespoon of olive oil in a large skillet over medium-high heat.
3. Add minced garlic and red pepper flakes (if using) to the skillet. Sauté for 1 minute until fragrant.
4. Add the shrimp to the skillet and cook for 2-3 minutes on each side until pink and opaque. Remove shrimp from the skillet and set aside.
5. In the same skillet, add the remaining 1 tablespoon of olive oil. Add the zucchini noodles and toss gently for 2-3 minutes until just tender.
6. Return the cooked shrimp to the skillet with the zucchini noodles.
7. Add lemon zest and juice to the skillet, stirring to combine all ingredients evenly.
8. Season with salt and pepper to taste.
9. Divide the Lemon Garlic Shrimp with Zucchini Noodles between two plates.
10. Garnish with freshly chopped parsley.
11. Serve immediately and enjoy your light and flavorful dinner!

Nutritional Information (per serving):

Calories: Approximately 220 kcal

Protein: 25g

Carbohydrates: 8g

Fiber: 2g

HEALTH BENEFITS:

Shrimp is a low-calorie protein source rich in selenium, vitamin B12, and iodine. Zucchini noodles are low in carbs and calories, providing a healthy and hydrating alternative to pasta. Lemon and garlic add antioxidants and anti-inflammatory benefits.

POINT VALUE:

5

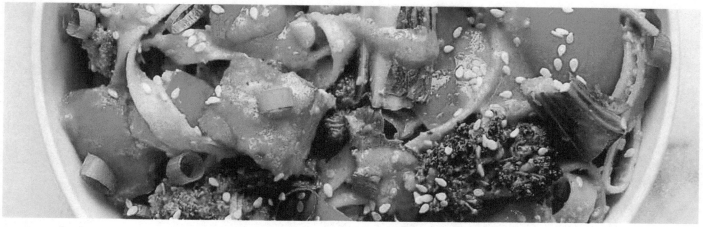

Veggie Stir-Fry with Tofu

COOKING TIME: 20 MIN | PREP TIME: 15 MIN | TOTAL TIME: 35 MIN | SERVING SIZE: 4

INGREDIENTS:

- 14 oz extra-firm tofu, drained and pressed
- 1 tablespoon cornstarch
- 2 tablespoons low-sodium soy sauce
- 1 tablespoon hoisin sauce
- 1 tablespoon sesame oil
- 1 tablespoon olive oil
- 1 bell pepper, thinly sliced
- 1 cup broccoli florets
- 1 cup snap peas
- 1 carrot, thinly sliced
- 2 cloves garlic, minced
- 1-inch piece of ginger, minced
- 2 green onions, chopped
- Salt and pepper to taste
- Cooked brown rice, Pasta or quinoa, for serving (optional, not included in points)

INSTRUCTIONS:

1. Cut the pressed tofu into cubes and toss them with cornstarch until evenly coated.
2. In a small bowl, mix together soy sauce and hoisin sauce. Set aside.
3. Heat olive oil in a large skillet or wok over medium-high heat. Add tofu cubes and cook until golden brown on all sides, about 5-7 minutes. Remove tofu from skillet and set aside.
4. In the same skillet, add sesame oil and sauté bell pepper, broccoli, snap peas, and carrot for 3-4 minutes until vegetables are tender-crisp.
5. Add minced garlic and ginger to the skillet and cook for 1 minute until fragrant.
6. Return the cooked tofu to the skillet. Pour the soy sauce mixture over the tofu and vegetables. Stir well to coat everything evenly.
7. Cook for another 2-3 minutes, stirring occasionally, until the sauce thickens slightly and everything is heated through.
8. Season with salt and pepper to taste. Garnish with chopped green onions.
9. Serve hot over cooked brown rice or quinoa if desired (note: brown rice or quinoa is optional and not included in the point value).

HEALTH BENEFITS:

Tofu is a plant-based protein that contains all nine essential amino acids. The mixed vegetables provide a variety of vitamins, minerals, and fiber, supporting overall health and digestion. This dish is low in calories but high in nutrients, making it ideal for weight loss.

Nutritional Information (per serving):
Calories: Approximately 220 kcal
Protein: 14g
Carbohydrates: 14g
Fiber: 4g

POINT VALUE:

4

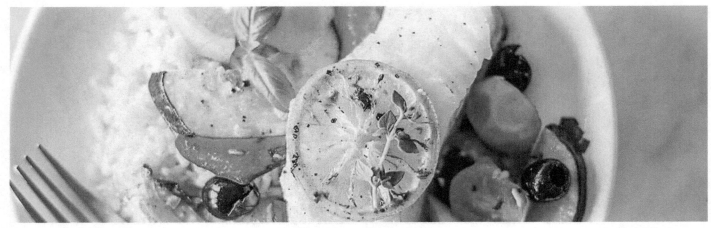

Baked Cod with Mediterranean Vegetables

COOKING TIME: 25 MIN | PREP TIME: 15 MIN | TOTAL TIME: 40 MIN | SERVING SIZE: 4

INGREDIENTS:

- 4 cod fillets (about 6 oz each)
- 2 cups cherry tomatoes, halved
- 1 medium red onion, thinly sliced
- 1 medium zucchini, sliced
- 1 medium yellow bell pepper, sliced
- 1/4 cup Kalamata olives, pitted and halved
- 2 tablespoons extra virgin olive oil
- 3 cloves garlic, minced
- 1 teaspoon dried oregano
- 1/2 teaspoon dried thyme
- Salt and pepper to taste
- Fresh parsley, chopped (for garnish)

INSTRUCTIONS:

1. Preheat your oven to 400°F (200°C). Line a baking sheet with parchment paper or lightly grease with olive oil.
2. In a large bowl, combine cherry tomatoes, red onion, zucchini, yellow bell pepper, and Kalamata olives. Drizzle with 1 tablespoon of olive oil and sprinkle with minced garlic, dried oregano, dried thyme, salt, and pepper. Toss to coat evenly.
3. Spread the vegetable mixture evenly on the prepared baking sheet. Bake in the preheated oven for 15-20 minutes, or until the vegetables are tender and starting to caramelize around the edges.
4. While the vegetables are baking, prepare the cod fillets. Pat dry the cod fillets with paper towels and place them on a separate baking sheet or oven-safe dish.
5. Drizzle the remaining 1 tablespoon of olive oil over the cod fillets. Season both sides of the cod fillets with salt and pepper.
6. Once the vegetables are done baking, remove the baking sheet from the oven and place the seasoned cod fillets on top of the vegetables.
7. Return the baking sheet to the oven and bake for an additional 10-12 minutes, or until the cod is cooked through and flakes easily with a fork.
8. Remove from the oven and let rest for a few minutes before serving.
9. Divide the Baked Cod with Mediterranean Vegetables among four plates. Garnish with chopped fresh parsley.
10. Serve hot and enjoy your flavorful and nutritious dinner!

HEALTH BENEFITS:

Cod is a lean protein that is low in fat and calories. Mediterranean vegetables, such as tomatoes, bell peppers, and olives, are rich in vitamins, antioxidants, and healthy fats. This combination supports heart health, reduces inflammation, and promotes weight loss.

POINT VALUE:

5

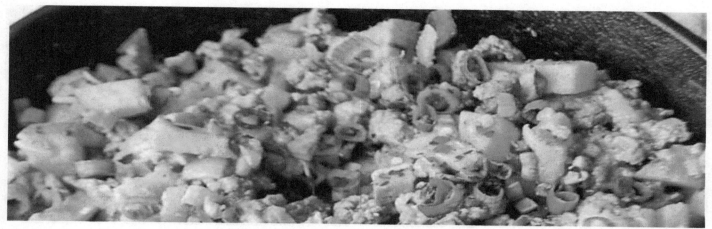

Turkey and Sweet Potato Skillet

COOKING TIME: 25 MIN | PREP TIME: 10 MIN | TOTAL TIME: 35 MIN | SERVING SIZE: 4

INGREDIENTS:

- 1 lb lean ground turkey
- 2 medium sweet potatoes, peeled and diced
- 1 bell pepper, diced (any color)
- 1 onion, diced
- 2 cloves garlic, minced
- 1 teaspoon paprika
- 1 teaspoon dried oregano
- 1/2 teaspoon ground cumin
- Salt and pepper to taste
- 1 tablespoon olive oil
- Fresh parsley or cilantro, chopped (for garnish, optional)

INSTRUCTIONS:

1. Heat olive oil in a large skillet over medium-high heat.
2. Add diced sweet potatoes to the skillet and cook for 5-7 minutes until they start to soften.
3. Push the sweet potatoes to the side of the skillet and add ground turkey to the empty space. Break up the turkey with a spatula and cook until browned and cooked through, about 5-7 minutes.
4. Stir in diced bell pepper, onion, and minced garlic. Cook for another 3-4 minutes until vegetables are tender.
5. Sprinkle paprika, dried oregano, ground cumin, salt, and pepper over the skillet. Stir well to combine all ingredients.
6. Reduce heat to medium-low and cover the skillet. Let it simmer for 5-7 minutes, stirring occasionally, until sweet potatoes are tender.
7. Taste and adjust seasoning if needed.
8. Remove from heat and garnish with fresh parsley or cilantro if desired.
9. Divide the Turkey and Sweet Potato Skillet into 4 servings and serve hot.

Nutritional Information (per serving):
Calories: Approximately 300 kcal
Protein: 25g
Carbohydrates: 20g
Fiber: 4g

HEALTH BENEFITS:
Ground turkey is a lean protein source, while sweet potatoes are high in fiber, vitamins A and C, and antioxidants. This dish supports immune function, provides energy, and helps keep you full longer, making it great for weight management.

POINT VALUE:

6

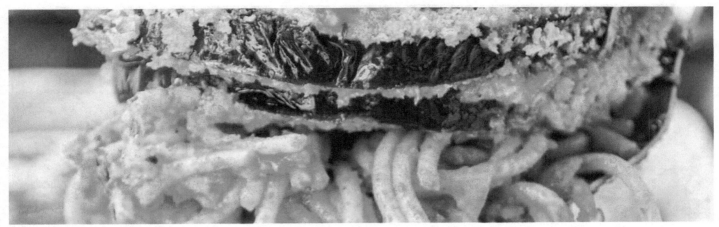

Eggplant Parmesan with Whole Wheat Pasta

COOKING TIME: 45 MIN | PREP TIME: 20 MIN | TOTAL TIME: 1 HR 5 MIN | SERVING SIZE: 4

INGREDIENTS:

- 1 medium eggplant, sliced into 1/2-inch rounds
- 1 cup whole wheat breadcrumbs
- 1/2 cup grated Parmesan cheese
- 2 eggs, lightly beaten
- 2 cups marinara sauce (store-bought or homemade)
- 8 oz whole wheat spaghetti or pasta of choice
- 1 cup shredded part-skim mozzarella cheese
- 1 tablespoon olive oil
- Salt and pepper to taste
- Fresh basil leaves for garnish (optional)

HEALTH BENEFITS:

Eggplant is low in calories and high in fiber and antioxidants. Whole wheat pasta provides complex carbohydrates and additional fiber, supporting sustained energy and digestive health. This lighter version of a classic dish offers the benefits of traditional flavors with fewer calories.

INSTRUCTIONS:

1. Preheat the oven to 400°F (200°C). Line a baking sheet with parchment paper or lightly grease with olive oil.
2. In a shallow bowl, combine whole wheat breadcrumbs and grated Parmesan cheese. Season with salt and pepper to taste.
3. Dip each eggplant slice into the beaten eggs, then coat both sides with the breadcrumb mixture. Place the coated eggplant slices on the prepared baking sheet.
4. Bake the eggplant slices in the preheated oven for 20-25 minutes, flipping halfway through, until golden brown and crispy.
5. While the eggplant is baking, cook the whole wheat pasta according to package instructions until al dente. Drain and set aside.
6. In a medium saucepan, heat olive oil over medium heat. Add marinara sauce and simmer for 5-7 minutes until heated through.
7. In a 9x13-inch baking dish, spread a thin layer of marinara sauce on the bottom. Arrange half of the baked eggplant slices over the sauce.
8. Spoon half of the remaining marinara sauce over the eggplant slices, then sprinkle half of the shredded mozzarella cheese on top.
9. Repeat with the remaining eggplant slices, marinara sauce, and shredded mozzarella cheese.
10. Bake the Eggplant Parmesan in the oven for 20-25 minutes, until the cheese is melted and bubbly.
11. Serve the Eggplant Parmesan hot over a portion of whole wheat pasta, garnished with fresh basil leaves if desired.

POINT VALUE:

5

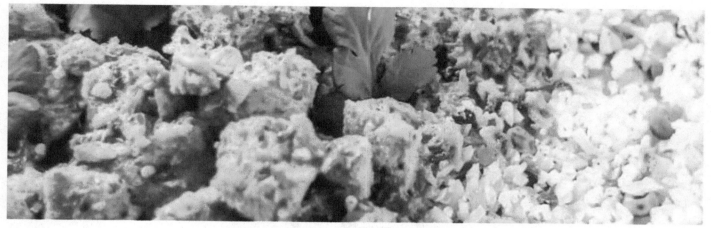

Coconut Curry Chicken with Cauliflower Rice

COOKING TIME: 25 MIN | PREP TIME: 15 MIN | TOTAL TIME: 40 MIN | SERVING SIZE: 4

INGREDIENTS:

- 1 ribeye steak (about 8-10 ounces)
- Salt an1 lb boneless, skinless chicken breasts, cut into bite-sized pieces
- 1 small head cauliflower, grated or finely chopped (about 4 cups)
- 1 can (14 oz) coconut milk (light version to reduce calories, if desired)
- 1 cup mixed vegetables (such as bell peppers, snap peas, carrots)
- 2 tablespoons red curry paste
- 2 cloves garlic, minced
- 1 tablespoon fresh ginger, grated
- 1 tablespoon olive oil
- Salt and pepper to taste
- Fresh cilantro, for garnish (optional)d pepper, to taste
- 2 tablespoons unsalted butter, at room temperature
- 1 tablespoon fresh parsley, finely chopped
- 1 clove garlic, minced

HEALTH BENEFITS:

Chicken provides lean protein, while cauliflower rice is a low-carb, low-calorie alternative to regular rice. Coconut milk adds healthy fats, and the curry spices offer anti-inflammatory and antioxidant benefits. This dish is flavorful and nutritious, supporting weight loss and overall health.

INSTRUCTIONS:

1. Heat olive oil in a large skillet or wok over medium-high heat. Add minced garlic and grated ginger, and sauté for 1-2 minutes until fragrant.
2. Add chicken pieces to the skillet and cook until browned on all sides, about 5-6 minutes.
3. Stir in red curry paste and mix well to coat the chicken.
4. Pour in coconut milk and bring to a simmer. Reduce heat to medium-low and let it simmer gently for 10-12 minutes until the chicken is cooked through and the sauce has thickened slightly.
5. Meanwhile, in a separate skillet, heat a little olive oil over medium heat. Add grated cauliflower and mixed vegetables. Sauté for 5-6 minutes until the cauliflower is tender-crisp.
6. Season the cauliflower rice and vegetables with salt and pepper to taste.
7. Divide the cauliflower rice and vegetables among serving plates.
8. Spoon the Coconut Curry Chicken over the cauliflower rice.
9. Garnish with fresh cilantro if desired.
10. Serve hot and enjoy your flavorful Coconut Curry Chicken with Cauliflower Rice!

Nutritional Information (per serving):

Calories: Approximately 380 kcal
Protein: 30g
Carbohydrates: 14g
Fiber: 5g

POINT VALUE:

6

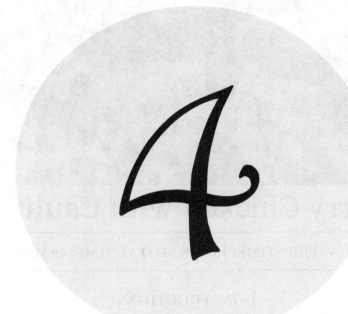

MAIN COURSE RECIPES

Welcome to the heart of our WATCH YOUR WEIGHT COOKBOOK – the Main Course Recipes. This section is designed to be the cornerstone of your daily meals, providing a delightful array of hearty and satisfying dishes that align perfectly with your weight loss goals.

Our main course recipes are crafted with a balance of lean proteins, wholesome grains, and vibrant vegetables, ensuring each meal is not only delicious but also nutritionally balanced. Whether you're in the mood for a comforting shepherd's pie or a light and refreshing stuffed pepper, each recipe has been thoughtfully designed to keep you full and energized without compromising on flavor.

Every recipe in this section comes with its point value clearly indicated, making it easier for you to stay on track with your weight management plan. These meals are versatile, easy to prepare, and perfect for both busy weeknights and leisurely weekend dinners. Embrace the joy of cooking and savor the benefits of nourishing your body with these delightful main course options.

Let's embark on this culinary journey together, one satisfying bite at a time!

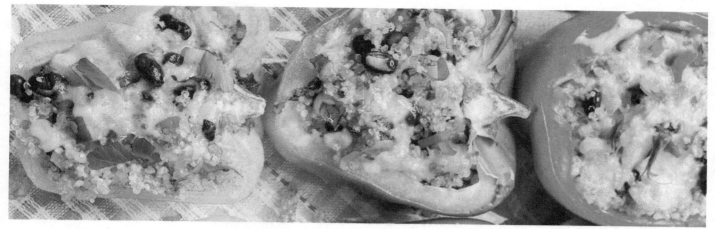

Quinoa and Black Bean Stuffed Peppers

COOKING TIME: 45 MIN | PREP TIME: 20 MIN | TOTAL TIME: 65 MIN | SERVING SIZE: 4

INGREDIENTS:

- 4 large bell peppers (any color), tops cut off and seeds removed
- 1 cup quinoa, rinsed
- 1 can (15 oz) black beans, drained and rinsed
- 1 cup corn kernels (fresh or frozen)
- 1 cup diced tomatoes (canned or fresh)
- 1/2 cup diced onion
- 2 cloves garlic, minced
- 1 teaspoon ground cumin
- 1/2 teaspoon chili powder
- Salt and pepper to taste
- 1 cup shredded low-fat cheese (such as cheddar or mozzarella)

INSTRUCTIONS:

1. Preheat the oven to 375°F (190°C). Grease a baking dish large enough to hold the bell peppers upright.
2. In a medium saucepan, bring 2 cups of water to a boil. Add quinoa, reduce heat to low, cover, and simmer for 15-20 minutes until quinoa is cooked and water is absorbed.
3. In a large skillet, heat olive oil over medium heat. Add diced onion and cook for 3-4 minutes until softened.
4. Add minced garlic, ground cumin, and chili powder to the skillet. Cook for 1-2 minutes until fragrant.
5. Stir in black beans, corn kernels, and diced tomatoes. Cook for another 5-6 minutes until heated through. Season with salt and pepper to taste.
6. Remove skillet from heat and stir in cooked quinoa until well combined.
7. Stuff each bell pepper with the quinoa and black bean mixture, packing it tightly.
8. Place stuffed peppers upright in the prepared baking dish.
9. Cover the dish with aluminum foil and bake in the preheated oven for 30-35 minutes, until the peppers are tender.
10. Remove foil, sprinkle shredded cheese evenly over the tops of the peppers, and return to the oven. Bake uncovered for another 5-10 minutes until the cheese is melted and bubbly.
11. Garnish with fresh cilantro if desired.
12. Serve hot and enjoy your nutritious and flavorful Quinoa and Black Bean Stuffed Peppers!

HEALTH BENEFITS:

Quinoa is a complete protein, providing all nine essential amino acids, and black beans are rich in fiber and protein. Bell peppers are high in vitamins A and C, which support immune function. This dish is nutrient-dense and promotes satiety, making it ideal for weight management.

POINT VALUE:

5

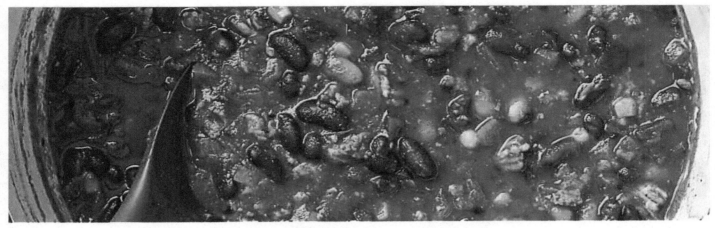

Turkey Chili with Beans

COOKING TIME: 30 MIN | PREP TIME: 15 MIN | TOTAL TIME: 45 MIN | SERVING SIZE: 6

INGREDIENTS:

- 1 lb lean ground turkey
- 1 onion, diced
- 2 cloves garlic, minced
- 1 bell pepper, diced (any color)
- 1 can (14 oz) diced tomatoes, undrained
- 1 can (15 oz) kidney beans, drained and rinsed
- 1 can (15 oz) black beans, drained and rinsed
- 1 cup low-sodium chicken broth
- 2 tablespoons tomato paste
- 1 tablespoon chili powder
- 1 teaspoon ground cumin
- 1/2 teaspoon paprika
- Salt and pepper to taste
- Fresh cilantro, for garnish (optional)

INSTRUCTIONS:

1. In a large pot or Dutch oven, heat olive oil over medium heat. Add diced onion, minced garlic, and diced bell pepper. Sauté for 3-4 minutes until vegetables are softened.
2. Add ground turkey to the pot and cook, breaking it apart with a spoon, until browned and cooked through, about 5-6 minutes.
3. Stir in chili powder, ground cumin, paprika, salt, and pepper. Cook for another 1-2 minutes until fragrant.
4. Add diced tomatoes, kidney beans, black beans, chicken broth, and tomato paste to the pot. Stir well to combine.
5. Bring the chili to a boil, then reduce heat to low. Simmer uncovered for 20-25 minutes, stirring occasionally, until the flavors have melded and the chili has thickened.
6. Taste and adjust seasoning with salt and pepper if needed.
7. Serve hot, garnished with fresh cilantro if desired.

Nutritional Information (per serving):

Calories: Approximately 280 kcal

Protein: 25g

Carbohydrates: 31g

Fiber: 10g

HEALTH BENEFITS:

Turkey is a lean protein that helps build and repair muscles. Beans are a great source of fiber, protein, and essential nutrients like iron and folate. This chili is hearty and filling, supporting weight loss by keeping you full longer.

POINT VALUE:

4

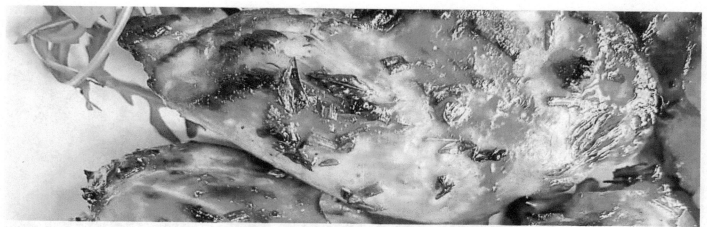

Baked Chicken Breast with Rosemary and Garlic

COOKING TIME: 25 MIN | PREP TIME: 10 MIN | TOTAL TIME: 35 MIN | SERVING SIZE: 4

INGREDIENTS:

- 4 boneless, skinless chicken breasts (about 1.5 lbs total)
- 4 cloves garlic, minced
- 2 tablespoons fresh rosemary, chopped
- 2 tablespoons olive oil
- Salt and pepper to taste
- Lemon wedges, for serving (optional)

INSTRUCTIONS:

1. Preheat your oven to 400°F (200°C).
2. In a small bowl, combine minced garlic, chopped rosemary, olive oil, salt, and pepper.
3. Pat the chicken breasts dry with paper towels and place them on a baking dish or sheet pan.
4. Rub the garlic and rosemary mixture evenly over both sides of the chicken breasts.
5. Bake in the preheated oven for 20-25 minutes, or until the chicken reaches an internal temperature of 165°F (75°C) and juices run clear.
6. Remove from the oven and let the chicken rest for a few minutes before serving.
7. Serve the Baked Chicken Breast with Rosemary and Garlic hot, optionally with lemon wedges on the side for extra flavor.

Nutritional Information (per serving):

Calories: Approximately 250 kcal

Protein: 30g

Carbohydrates: 1g

Fiber: 0g

HEALTH BENEFITS:

Chicken breast is a lean source of high-quality protein. Rosemary and garlic add antioxidants and anti-inflammatory properties without adding extra calories. This dish is simple, nutritious, and perfect for a weight loss-friendly meal.

POINT VALUE:

4

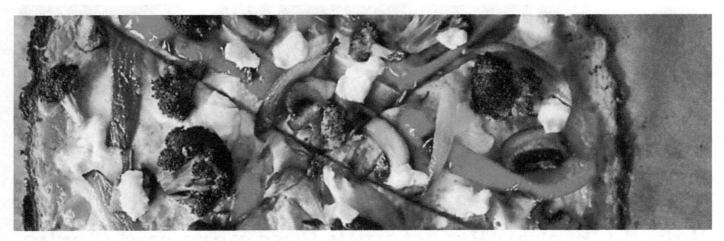

Cauliflower Crust Pizza with Veggies

COOKING TIME: 30 MIN | PREP TIME: 20 MIN | TOTAL TIME: 50 MIN | SERVING SIZE: 2

INGREDIENTS:

- 1 small head cauliflower, grated (about 4 cups)
- 1/2 cup shredded mozzarella cheese
- 1/4 cup grated Parmesan cheese
- 1 teaspoon dried oregano
- 1/2 teaspoon garlic powder
- 1/4 teaspoon salt
- 1/4 teaspoon black pepper
- 1 egg, beaten
- 1/2 cup tomato sauce (no sugar added)
- 1 cup mixed vegetables (such as bell peppers, mushrooms, onions, spinach)
- 1/2 cup shredded part-skim mozzarella cheese

POINT VALUE:

6

HEALTH BENEFITS:

Cauliflower crust is a low-carb alternative to traditional pizza crust, reducing calorie intake. The variety of veggies adds vitamins, minerals, and fiber, supporting overall health and digestion. This pizza is a delicious and healthier way to enjoy a favorite dish.

INSTRUCTIONS:

1. Preheat your oven to 400°F (200°C). Line a baking sheet with parchment paper.
2. Grate the cauliflower using a box grater or food processor until it resembles rice.
3. Place the grated cauliflower in a microwave-safe bowl and microwave on high for 5-6 minutes, or until softened. Let it cool slightly.
4. Transfer the cooked cauliflower to a clean kitchen towel or cheesecloth. Squeeze out as much moisture as possible. This step is crucial for a crispy crust.
5. In a mixing bowl, combine the squeezed cauliflower, shredded mozzarella cheese, Parmesan cheese, dried oregano, garlic powder, salt, pepper, and beaten egg. Mix until well combined.
6. Transfer the cauliflower mixture onto the prepared baking sheet. Use your hands to press it into a round pizza crust shape, about 1/4-inch thick.
7. Bake the cauliflower crust in the preheated oven for 20-25 minutes, or until golden brown and firm to the touch.
8. While the crust is baking, prepare your toppings. Spread tomato sauce evenly over the baked crust, leaving a small border around the edges.
9. Top with mixed vegetables and sprinkle shredded part-skim mozzarella cheese over the pizza.
10. Return the pizza to the oven and bake for an additional 10-12 minutes, or until the cheese is melted and bubbly.
11. Remove from the oven and let it cool for a few minutes before slicing.
12. Serve hot and enjoy your delicious Cauliflower Crust Pizza with Veggies!

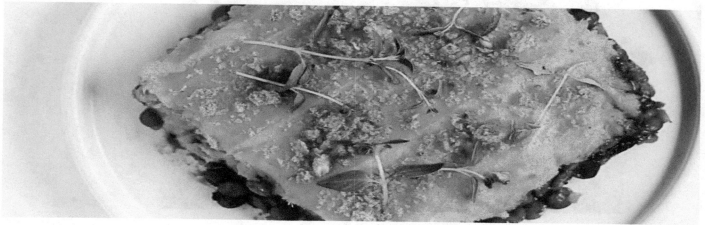

Lentil and Sweet Potato Shepherd's Pie

COOKING TIME: 45 MIN | PREP TIME: 20 MIN | TOTAL TIME: 65 MIN | SERVING SIZE: 6

INGREDIENTS:

- 2 large sweet potatoes, peeled and cubed
- 1 cup dry green or brown lentils
- 2 cups vegetable broth
- 1 tablespoon olive oil
- 1 onion, chopped
- 2 cloves garlic, minced
- 2 carrots, diced
- 2 celery stalks, diced
- 1 cup frozen peas
- 1 tablespoon tomato paste
- 1 teaspoon dried thyme
- 1 teaspoon dried rosemary
- Salt and pepper to taste

INSTRUCTIONS:

1. Preheat oven to 400°F (200°C).
2. Place sweet potatoes in a large pot, cover with water, and bring to a boil. Cook until tender, about 15-20 minutes. Drain and mash with a fork or potato masher until smooth. Set aside.
3. In a separate pot, combine lentils and vegetable broth. Bring to a boil, then reduce heat and simmer for 20-25 minutes until lentils are tender and most of the liquid is absorbed. Drain any excess liquid and set aside.
4. In a large skillet, heat olive oil over medium heat. Add chopped onion, garlic, carrots, and celery. Sauté for 5-7 minutes until vegetables are softened.
5. Stir in tomato paste, dried thyme, dried rosemary, salt, and pepper. Cook for 1-2 minutes until fragrant.
6. Add cooked lentils and frozen peas to the skillet. Stir well to combine all ingredients. Cook for another 2-3 minutes until heated through.
7. Transfer the lentil and vegetable mixture to a baking dish. Spread mashed sweet potatoes evenly over the top.
8. Place the baking dish in the preheated oven and bake for 20-25 minutes until the sweet potato topping is lightly golden.
9. Remove from oven and let cool for a few minutes before serving.
10. Serve hot and enjoy your comforting and nutritious Lentil and Sweet Potato Shepherd's Pie!

HEALTH BENEFITS:

Lentils are rich in protein, fiber, and essential nutrients like iron and folate. Sweet potatoes provide vitamins A and C, potassium, and antioxidants. This dish is filling and nutritious, promoting satiety and supporting weight loss goals.

POINT VALUE:

5

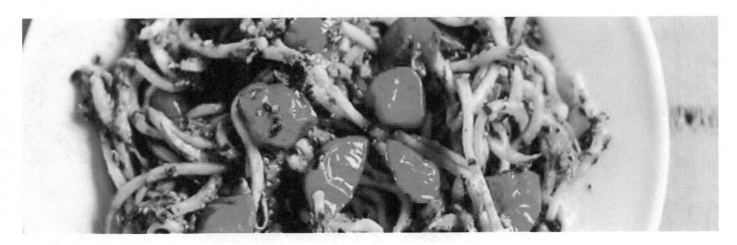

Zucchini Noodles with Pesto and Cherry Tomatoes

COOKING TIME: 10 MIN | PREP TIME: 10 MIN | TOTAL TIME: 20 MIN | SERVING SIZE: 2

INGREDIENTS:

- 2 medium zucchini
- 1 cup cherry tomatoes, halved
- 2 tablespoons prepared basil pesto
- 2 tablespoons grated Parmesan cheese
- 1 tablespoon olive oil
- Salt and pepper to taste
- Fresh basil leaves, for garnish (optional)

INSTRUCTIONS:

1. Using a spiralizer or vegetable peeler, create zucchini noodles (zoodles) from the zucchini. Set aside.
2. Heat olive oil in a large skillet over medium heat. Add cherry tomatoes and sauté for 2-3 minutes until they start to soften.
3. Add zucchini noodles to the skillet and toss with the cherry tomatoes.
4. Cook the zucchini noodles for 3-4 minutes, stirring occasionally, until they are just tender but still crisp.
5. Stir in basil pesto and mix well to coat the zucchini noodles evenly.
6. Remove the skillet from heat and season with salt and pepper to taste.
7. Divide the zucchini noodles with pesto and cherry tomatoes between serving plates.
8. Sprinkle grated Parmesan cheese over each serving.
9. Garnish with fresh basil leaves if desired.
10. Serve immediately and enjoy your delicious and low-calorie Zucchini Noodles with Pesto and Cherry Tomatoes!

Nutritional Information (per serving):
Calories: Approximately 180 kcal
Protein: 5g
Carbohydrates: 10g
Fiber: 3g

HEALTH BENEFITS:
Zucchini noodles are low in calories and carbs, making them a healthy alternative to pasta. Pesto adds healthy fats from nuts and olive oil, while cherry tomatoes provide vitamins and antioxidants. This dish is light, flavorful, and ideal for weight management.

POINT VALUE:

4

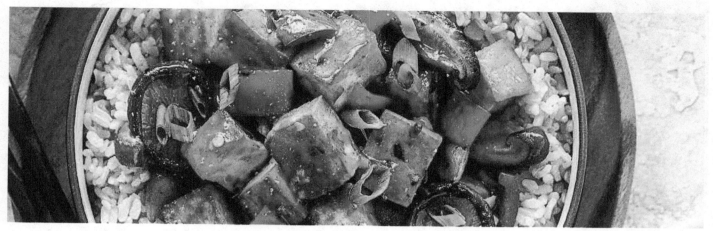

Spicy Tofu Stir-Fry with Brown Rice

COOKING TIME: 20 MIN | PREP TIME: 15 MIN | TOTAL TIME: 35 MIN | SERVING SIZE: 4

INGREDIENTS:

- 1 block (14 oz) extra-firm tofu, drained and pressed
- 2 cups cooked brown rice
- 1 cup mixed vegetables (such as bell peppers, broccoli, snap peas)
- 1 red chili pepper, thinly sliced
- 2 cloves garlic, minced
- 1 tablespoon fresh ginger, grated
- 3 tablespoons low-sodium soy sauce
- 1 tablespoon rice vinegar
- 1 tablespoon sesame oil
- 1 tablespoon olive oil
- Fresh cilantro, for garnish (optional)
- Sesame seeds, for garnish (optional)

INSTRUCTIONS:

1. Cut the pressed tofu into cubes or rectangles.
2. Heat olive oil in a large skillet or wok over medium-high heat. Add minced garlic, grated ginger, and sliced red chili pepper. Sauté for 1-2 minutes until fragrant.
3. Add tofu cubes to the skillet and cook for 5-6 minutes, stirring occasionally, until lightly browned on all sides.
4. Stir in mixed vegetables and continue to cook for another 3-4 minutes until vegetables are tender-crisp.
5. In a small bowl, mix together soy sauce, rice vinegar, and sesame oil.
6. Pour the sauce mixture over the tofu and vegetables in the skillet. Stir well to coat evenly.
7. Cook for another 2-3 minutes, allowing the sauce to thicken slightly and flavors to meld together.
8. Divide the cooked brown rice among serving plates.
9. Spoon the Spicy Tofu Stir-Fry over the brown rice.
10. Garnish with fresh cilantro and sesame seeds if desired.
11. Serve hot and enjoy your flavorful Spicy Tofu Stir-Fry with Brown Rice!

Nutritional Information (per serving):

Calories: Approximately 320 kcal

Protein: 15g

Carbohydrates: 35g

Fiber: 5g

POINT VALUE:

5

HEALTH BENEFITS:

Tofu is a plant-based protein that contains all essential amino acids. Brown rice is a whole grain that provides fiber and sustained energy. The mixed vegetables add a range of vitamins and minerals. This stir-fry is nutrient-dense and supports overall health and weight loss.

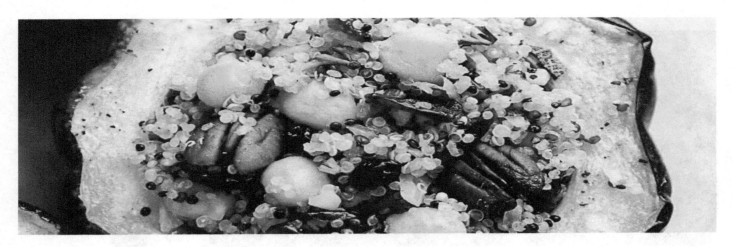

Stuffed Acorn Squash with Quinoa and Cranberries

COOKING TIME: 50 MIN | PREP TIME: 15 MIN | TOTAL TIME: 1 HR 5 MIN | SERVING SIZE: 4

INGREDIENTS:

- 2 acorn squash, halved and seeds removed
- 1 cup quinoa, rinsed
- 2 cups vegetable broth or water
- 1/2 cup dried cranberries
- 1/2 cup chopped pecans or walnuts
- 1/4 cup chopped fresh parsley
- 2 tablespoons olive oil
- 1 onion, diced
- 2 cloves garlic, minced
- 1 teaspoon ground cinnamon
- Salt and pepper to taste

HEALTH BENEFITS:

Acorn squash is rich in vitamins A and C, potassium, and fiber. Quinoa is a complete protein, and cranberries add antioxidants and a touch of sweetness. This dish is both nutritious and satisfying, promoting satiety and supporting weight management.

INSTRUCTIONS:

1. Preheat the oven to 400°F (200°C).
2. Place the acorn squash halves cut-side down on a baking sheet lined with parchment paper. Bake for 30-35 minutes, or until the squash is tender when pierced with a fork.
3. While the squash is baking, rinse the quinoa under cold water and drain well.
4. In a medium saucepan, bring the vegetable broth (or water) to a boil. Add the quinoa, reduce heat to low, cover, and simmer for 15 minutes, or until the liquid is absorbed and the quinoa is fluffy.
5. In a large skillet, heat olive oil over medium heat. Add diced onion and garlic, and sauté until softened and fragrant, about 3-4 minutes.
6. Add cooked quinoa to the skillet with onions and garlic. Stir in dried cranberries, chopped nuts, chopped parsley, ground cinnamon, salt, and pepper. Mix well to combine all ingredients.
7. Remove the baked acorn squash halves from the oven. Carefully flip them over using tongs or a spatula.
8. Divide the quinoa mixture evenly among the acorn squash halves, packing it lightly into each cavity.
9. Return the stuffed acorn squash to the oven and bake for an additional 15 minutes, or until the tops are lightly browned.
10. Remove from the oven and let cool slightly before serving.
11. Garnish with additional chopped parsley if desired.
12. Serve hot and enjoy your nutritious and flavorful Stuffed Acorn Squash with Quinoa and Cranberries!

POINT VALUE:

6

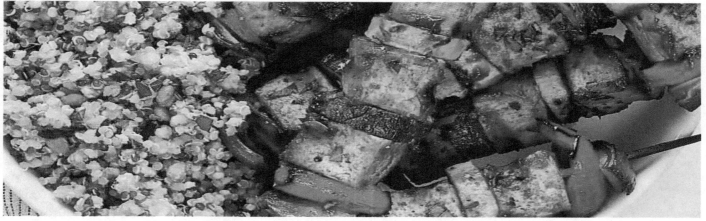

Grilled Veggie Skewers with Quinoa

COOKING TIME: 20 MIN | PREP TIME: 15 MIN | TOTAL TIME: 35 MIN | SERVING SIZE: 4

INGREDIENTS:

- 1 cup quinoa, uncooked
- 2 cups water or vegetable broth
- 1 red bell pepper, cut into chunks
- 1 yellow bell pepper, cut into chunks
- 1 zucchini, sliced into rounds
- 1 yellow squash, sliced into rounds
- 1 red onion, cut into chunks
- 8-10 cherry tomatoes
- 8-10 button mushrooms
- 2 tablespoons olive oil
- 2 tablespoons balsamic vinegar
- 2 cloves garlic, minced
- 1 teaspoon dried oregano
- Salt and pepper to taste
- Fresh parsley or basil, for garnish (optional)

INSTRUCTIONS:

1. Rinse the quinoa under cold water to remove any bitterness. In a medium saucepan, bring 2 cups of water or vegetable broth to a boil. Add the quinoa, reduce heat to low, cover, and simmer for 15-20 minutes until the quinoa is cooked and liquid is absorbed. Fluff with a fork and set aside.
2. While the quinoa is cooking, prepare the vegetables for skewering. In a large bowl, combine the bell peppers, zucchini, yellow squash, red onion, cherry tomatoes, and mushrooms.
3. In a small bowl, whisk together olive oil, balsamic vinegar, minced garlic, dried oregano, salt, and pepper.
4. Pour the marinade over the vegetables and toss gently to coat. Let marinate for 10-15 minutes.
5. Preheat the grill or grill pan over medium-high heat. Thread the marinated vegetables onto skewers, alternating between different vegetables.
6. Grill the veggie skewers for 8-10 minutes, turning occasionally, until the vegetables are tender and lightly charred.
7. Serve the grilled veggie skewers over a bed of cooked quinoa.
8. Garnish with fresh parsley or basil if desired.
9. Enjoy your nutritious and delicious Grilled Veggie Skewers with Quinoa!

HEALTH BENEFITS:

Grilled veggies are low in calories but high in vitamins, minerals, and antioxidants. Quinoa provides complete protein and fiber, making this dish a balanced and filling meal. It's perfect for supporting weight loss while enjoying a variety of flavors.

POINT VALUE:

4

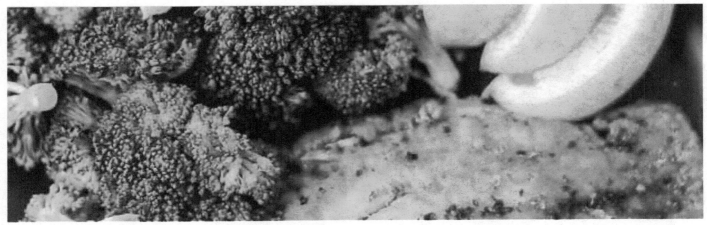

Lemon Herb Tilapia with Steamed Broccoli

COOKING TIME: 15 MIN | PREP TIME: 10 MIN | TOTAL TIME: 25 MIN | SERVING SIZE: 4

INGREDIENTS:

- 4 tilapia fillets (about 4-6 oz each)
- 1 lemon, thinly sliced
- 2 tablespoons fresh lemon juice
- 2 tablespoons olive oil
- 2 cloves garlic, minced
- 1 teaspoon dried thyme
- 1 teaspoon dried rosemary
- Salt and pepper to taste
- 4 cups broccoli florets

INSTRUCTIONS:

1. Preheat your oven to 400°F (200°C).
2. In a small bowl, mix together olive oil, minced garlic, dried thyme, dried rosemary, and fresh lemon juice.
3. Place tilapia fillets on a baking sheet lined with parchment paper. Season both sides of the tilapia fillets with salt and pepper.
4. Brush the herb and lemon mixture over each tilapia fillet.
5. Arrange lemon slices on top of the tilapia fillets.
6. Bake in the preheated oven for 12-15 minutes, or until the fish is opaque and flakes easily with a fork.
7. While the tilapia is baking, steam the broccoli florets until tender-crisp, about 5-6 minutes.
8. Divide the steamed broccoli among serving plates.
9. Place one tilapia fillet on top of each serving of steamed broccoli.
10. Serve hot, garnished with additional lemon slices if desired.
11. Enjoy your nutritious and delicious Lemon Herb Tilapia with Steamed Broccoli!

Nutritional Information (per serving):

Calories: Approximately 220 kcal

Protein: 26g

Carbohydrates: 6g

Fiber: 2g

HEALTH BENEFITS:

Tilapia is a lean source of protein, and broccoli is rich in vitamins C and K, fiber, and antioxidants. Lemon and herbs add flavor without extra calories. This dish is light, nutritious, and ideal for maintaining a healthy weight.

POINT VALUE:

5

5

GUILT-FREE DESSERT

Indulging in dessert doesn't have to derail your weight loss goals. In fact, enjoying a sweet treat can be a delightful and satisfying part of a balanced diet, especially when you choose recipes designed with your health in mind. Our Guilt-Free Dessert Recipes section is here to prove that you can have your cake and eat it too. Literally!

Each dessert in this collection is crafted to be lower in calories, sugars, and unhealthy fats, without compromising on taste or enjoyment. Whether you're craving something fruity, creamy, or chocolaty, you'll find a variety of options to satisfy your sweet tooth while keeping your health goals on track. From Mixed Berry Frozen Yogurt to Dark Chocolate Avocado Mousse, these recipes are not only delicious but also provide nutritional benefits that support your well-being.

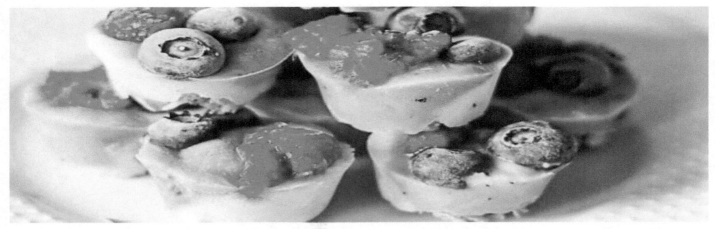

Mixed Berry Frozen Yogurt

COOKING TIME: 0 MIN | PREP TIME: 10 MIN | TOTAL TIME: 10 MIN | SERVING SIZE: 4

INGREDIENTS:

- 2 cups plain non-fat Greek yogurt
- 2 cups mixed berries (such as strawberries, blueberries, raspberries)
- 1-2 tablespoons honey or agave syrup (optional, not included in points)

INSTRUCTIONS:

1. In a blender or food processor, combine the Greek yogurt and mixed berries.
2. Blend until smooth and well combined.
3. Taste the mixture and add honey or agave syrup if desired, adjusting sweetness to your preference (note: honey or agave syrup is optional and not included in the point value).
4. Pour the yogurt mixture into a shallow, freezer-safe container.
5. Spread the mixture evenly with a spatula.
6. Cover the container with plastic wrap or a lid.
7. Place the container in the freezer and freeze for at least 4 hours, or until firm.
8. Once frozen, remove the container from the freezer and let the frozen yogurt sit at room temperature for a few minutes to soften slightly before serving.
9. Scoop the Mixed Berry Frozen Yogurt into serving bowls or cones.
10. Serve immediately and enjoy your refreshing and guilt-free dessert!

Nutritional Information (per serving):

Calories: Approximately 120 kcal

Protein: 12g

Carbohydrates: 16g

Fiber: 2g

HEALTH BENEFITS:

This dessert combines the probiotics and protein of Greek yogurt with the antioxidants, vitamins, and fiber of mixed berries. It's a low-calorie, nutritious treat that supports digestive health and satisfies your sweet tooth without compromising your weight loss goals.

POINT VALUE:

3

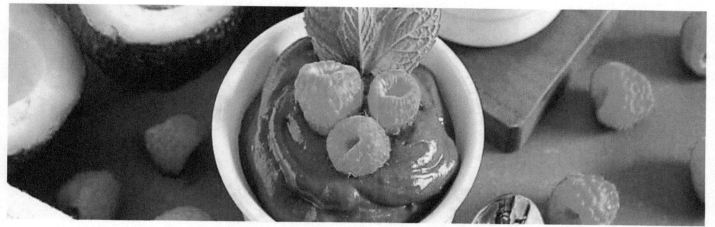

Dark Chocolate Avocado Mousse

COOKING TIME: 0 MIN | PREP TIME: 10 MIN | TOTAL TIME: 10 MIN | SERVING SIZE: 4

INGREDIENTS:

- 2 ripe avocados, peeled and pitted
- 1/4 cup unsweetened cocoa powder
- 1/4 cup honey or agave nectar (adjust sweetness to taste, not included in points)
- 1 teaspoon vanilla extract
- Pinch of salt
- 1/4 cup almond milk (or any milk of choice)
- Fresh berries, for garnish (optional, not included in points)

INSTRUCTIONS:

1. In a food processor or blender, combine the peeled and pitted avocados, unsweetened cocoa powder, honey or agave nectar (if using), and vanilla extract, pinch of salt, and almond milk.
2. Blend until smooth and creamy, scraping down the sides of the processor or blender as needed to ensure all ingredients are well combined.
3. Taste and adjust sweetness if necessary by adding more honey or agave nectar.
4. Divide the chocolate avocado mousse into serving dishes or glasses.
5. Cover and refrigerate for at least 1 hour to chill and firm up the mousse.
6. Before serving, garnish with fresh berries if desired.
7. Serve chilled and enjoy your indulgent yet healthy Dark Chocolate Avocado Mousse!

Nutritional Information (per serving):

Calories: Approximately 200 kcal

Protein: 3g

Carbohydrates: 20g

Fiber: 7g

HEALTH BENEFITS:

Avocados provide healthy monounsaturated fats, fiber, and essential vitamins like E and K. Dark chocolate is rich in antioxidants and may help improve heart health. This creamy dessert is both indulgent and nutritious, making it a smart choice for a guilt-free treat.

POINT VALUE:

4

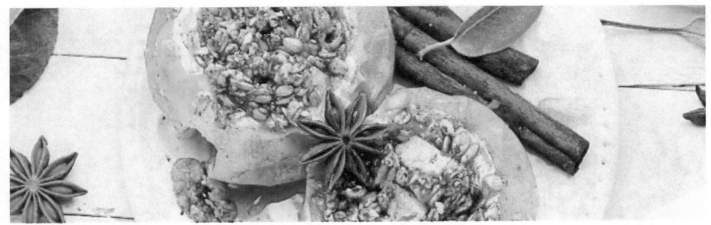

Baked Apple with Cinnamon and Walnuts

COOKING TIME: 30 MIN | PREP TIME: 10 MIN | TOTAL TIME: 40 MIN | SERVING SIZE: 1

INGREDIENTS:

- 1 medium apple (such as Granny Smith or Honey crisp)
- 1 tablespoon chopped walnuts
- 1 teaspoon honey (optional, not included in points)
- 1/2 teaspoon ground cinnamon

INSTRUCTIONS:

1. Preheat your oven to 375°F (190°C).
2. Wash and core the apple, removing the seeds and stem but leaving the bottom intact to hold the filling.
3. In a small bowl, mix together chopped walnuts and ground cinnamon.
4. Stuff the cored apple with the walnut and cinnamon mixture.
5. Place the stuffed apple on a baking sheet lined with parchment paper.
6. Bake in the preheated oven for 25-30 minutes, or until the apple is tender and the filling is golden brown.
7. Remove from the oven and let it cool slightly.
8. Drizzle with 1 teaspoon of honey if desired (note: honey is optional and not included in the point value).
9. Serve warm and enjoy your delightful Baked Apple with Cinnamon and Walnuts!

Nutritional Information (per serving):
Calories: Approximately 120 kcal
Protein: 1g
Carbohydrates: 20g
Fiber: 4g

HEALTH BENEFITS:
Apples are high in fiber and vitamin C, while cinnamon helps regulate blood sugar levels. Walnuts add healthy omega-3 fats, protein, and additional fiber. This dessert is comforting and wholesome, promoting satiety and supporting heart health.

POINT VALUE:

3

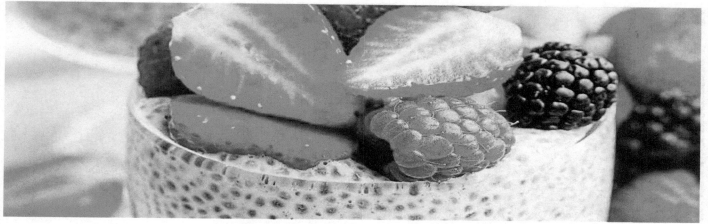

Chia Seed Pudding with Fresh Fruit

COOKING TIME: 0 MIN | PREP TIME: 5 MIN | TOTAL TIME: 4 HRS | SERVING SIZE: 1

INGREDIENTS:

- 2 tablespoons chia seeds
- 1/2 cup unsweetened almond milk (or any preferred milk)
- 1/2 teaspoon vanilla extract
- 1 teaspoon honey (optional, not included in points)
- 1/2 cup mixed fresh berries (such as strawberries, blueberries, raspberries)
- Fresh mint leaves for garnish (optional)

INSTRUCTIONS:

1. In a bowl or container with a lid, combine chia seeds, unsweetened almond milk, and vanilla extract. Stir well to mix thoroughly.
2. Cover the bowl or container and refrigerate for at least 4 hours or overnight, allowing the chia seeds to absorb the liquid and thicken into a pudding-like consistency.
3. Once the chia seed mixture has thickened, remove it from the refrigerator.
4. Stir the pudding to ensure it's well combined and creamy.
5. Transfer the chia seed pudding into a serving bowl or glass.
6. Top the pudding with mixed fresh berries.
7. Drizzle 1 teaspoon of honey over the pudding if desired (note: honey is optional and not included in the point value).
8. Garnish with fresh mint leaves for an extra touch of freshness and presentation.
9. Serve chilled and enjoy your delightful Chia Seed Pudding with Fresh Fruit!

Nutritional Information (per serving):
Calories: Approximately 160 kcal
Protein: 5g
Carbohydrates: 18g
Fiber: 10g

HEALTH BENEFITS:

Chia seeds are a powerhouse of omega-3 fatty acids, fiber, and protein. Fresh fruit adds vitamins, minerals, and natural sweetness. This pudding is a nutrient-dense option that aids in digestion and keeps you full longer, supporting weight management.

POINT VALUE:

3

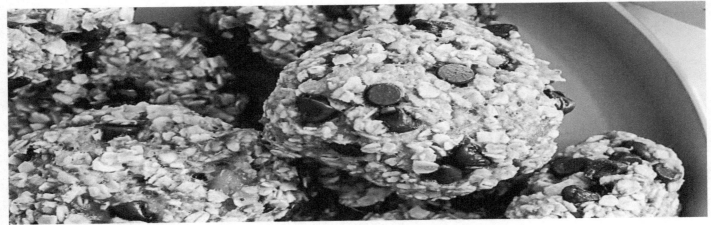

Banana Oatmeal Cookies

COOKING TIME: 15 MIN | PREP TIME: 10 MIN | TOTAL TIME: 25 MIN | SERVING SIZE: 12

INGREDIENTS:

- 2 ripe bananas, mashed
- 1 cup rolled oats
- 1/4 cup unsweetened applesauce
- 1/4 cup raisins
- 1/4 cup chopped walnuts
- 1 teaspoon vanilla extract
- 1/2 teaspoon ground cinnamon
- Pinch of salt

INSTRUCTIONS:

1. Preheat your oven to 350°F (175°C). Line a baking sheet with parchment paper.
2. In a large mixing bowl, mash the ripe bananas until smooth.
3. Add rolled oats, unsweetened applesauce, raisins, chopped walnuts, vanilla extract, ground cinnamon, and a pinch of salt to the bowl with the mashed bananas.
4. Stir all ingredients together until well combined and the mixture forms a sticky dough.
5. Scoop tablespoon-sized portions of the dough and place them onto the prepared baking sheet, spacing them evenly apart.
6. Flatten each cookie slightly with the back of a spoon or your fingers.
7. Bake in the preheated oven for 12-15 minutes, or until the cookies are lightly golden brown around the edges.
8. Remove from the oven and let the cookies cool on the baking sheet for 5 minutes before transferring them to a wire rack to cool completely.
9. Once cooled, store the Banana Oatmeal Cookies in an airtight container.
10. Enjoy your guilt-free and delicious Banana Oatmeal Cookies as a satisfying dessert option!

Nutritional Information (per cookie):
Calories: Approximately 70 kcal
Protein: 1.5g
Carbohydrates: 12g
Fiber: 1.5g

HEALTH BENEFITS:

Bananas are rich in potassium and fiber, while oats provide additional fiber and protein. These cookies are naturally sweetened and low in added sugars, making them a healthy and satisfying treat that can help maintain energy levels and support digestive health.

POINT VALUE:

3

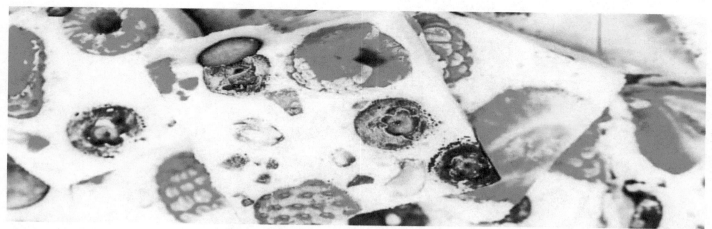

Greek Yogurt Bark with Berries and Almonds

COOKING TIME: 0 MIN | PREP TIME: 10 MIN | TOTAL TIME: 2 HRS 10 MIN | SERVING SIZE: 6

INGREDIENTS:

- 2 cups plain Greek yogurt (non-fat or low-fat)
- 1 tablespoon honey
- 1/2 cup mixed berries (such as strawberries, blueberries, raspberries), chopped if large
- 1/4 cup sliced almonds
- Zest of 1 lemon (optional, not included in points)

INSTRUCTIONS:

1. Line a baking sheet or large dish with parchment paper.
2. In a mixing bowl, combine Greek yogurt and honey. Stir until well combined.
3. Spread the Greek yogurt mixture evenly onto the lined baking sheet, about 1/4 inch thick.
4. Sprinkle chopped mixed berries and sliced almonds evenly over the Greek yogurt layer.
5. If using, sprinkle lemon zest over the top for additional flavor (optional).
6. Place the baking sheet in the freezer and freeze for at least 2 hours, or until the yogurt bark is completely firm.
7. Once frozen, remove the baking sheet from the freezer and break the bark into pieces using your hands or a knife.
8. Serve immediately as a refreshing dessert or snack.
9. Store any leftover Greek Yogurt Bark in an airtight container in the freezer.

Nutritional Information (per serving):

Calories: Approximately 110 kcal

Protein: 8g

Carbohydrates: 10g

Fiber: 1.5g

HEALTH BENEFITS:

Greek yogurt offers protein and probiotics, while berries contribute antioxidants and fiber. Almonds provide healthy fats and additional protein. This frozen treat is refreshing, nutritious, and helps support a healthy metabolism and digestive system.

POINT VALUE:

4

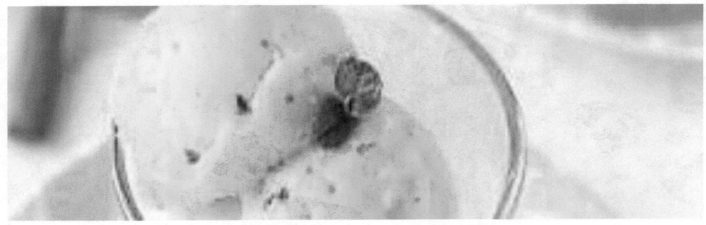

Mango Sorbet with Mint

COOKING TIME: 0 MIN | PREP TIME: 10 MIN | TOTAL TIME: 4 HRS | SERVING SIZE: 4

INGREDIENTS:

- 2 ripe mangoes, peeled and diced (about 2 cups)
- 1/4 cup fresh mint leaves, chopped
- 1 tablespoon fresh lime juice
- 1/4 cup water
- 2 tablespoons honey (optional, not included in points)

INSTRUCTIONS:

1. Place diced mangoes, chopped mint leaves, fresh lime juice, and water in a blender or food processor.
2. Blend until smooth and creamy.
3. Taste the mixture and add honey if desired for extra sweetness (note: honey is optional and not included in the point value).
4. Pour the mango mixture into a shallow, freezer-safe container.
5. Cover the container and place it in the freezer for at least 4 hours, or until the sorbet is firm.
6. Once the sorbet is frozen, scoop it into serving bowls or glasses.
7. Garnish with additional mint leaves if desired.
8. Serve immediately and enjoy your refreshing Mango Sorbet with Mint!

Nutritional Information (per serving):
Calories: Approximately 90 kcal
Protein: 1g
Carbohydrates: 23g
Fiber: 2g

HEALTH BENEFITS:
Mangoes are rich in vitamins A and C, fiber, and antioxidants. Mint adds a fresh flavor and aids in digestion. This sorbet is a low-calorie, hydrating dessert that satisfies your sweet cravings while providing essential nutrients and supporting weight loss.

POINT VALUE:

3

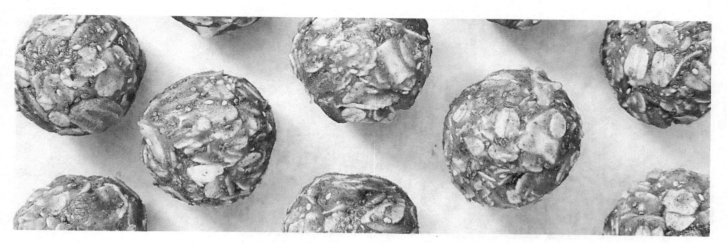

Pumpkin Spice Energy Balls

COOKING TIME: 0 MIN | PREP TIME: 15 MIN | TOTAL TIME: 15 MIN | SERVING SIZE: 12

INGREDIENTS:

- 1 cup rolled oats
- 1/2 cup pumpkin puree
- 1/4 cup almond butter
- 1/4 cup honey
- 1 teaspoon vanilla extract
- 1 teaspoon pumpkin pie spice
- 1/4 cup mini chocolate chips (optional, not included in point value)

INSTRUCTIONS:

1. In a large mixing bowl, combine rolled oats, pumpkin puree, almond butter, honey, vanilla extract, and pumpkin pie spice.
2. Mix well until all ingredients are thoroughly combined and form a sticky dough.
3. If using, gently fold in mini chocolate chips.
4. Using clean hands, scoop out about 1 tablespoon of the mixture and roll it into a ball between your palms. Repeat with the remaining mixture to form approximately 12 balls.
5. Place the energy balls on a plate or baking sheet lined with parchment paper.
6. Refrigerate the energy balls for at least 30 minutes to allow them to firm up.
7. Once chilled, transfer the energy balls to an airtight container and store in the refrigerator for up to one week.
8. Enjoy your delicious and nutritious Pumpkin Spice Energy Balls as a guilt-free dessert or snack!

Nutritional Information (per ball):

Calories: Approximately 90 kcal

Protein: 2g

Carbohydrates: 14g

Fiber: 2g

HEALTH BENEFITS:

Pumpkin is high in vitamins A and C, fiber, and antioxidants. These energy balls also contain healthy fats and protein from nuts or seeds, making them a nutritious and satisfying snack or dessert that can help maintain energy levels and support weight management.

POINT VALUE:

3

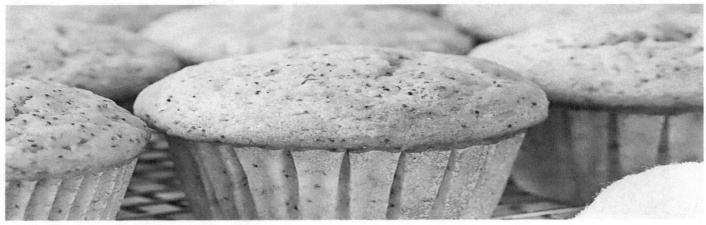

Almond Flour Lemon Poppy Seed Muffins

COOKING TIME: 20 MIN | PREP TIME: 15 MIN | TOTAL TIME: 35 MIN | SERVING SIZE: 12

INGREDIENTS:

- 2 cups almond flour
- 1/4 cup coconut flour
- 1/3 cup honey
- 1/4 cup melted coconut oil
- 3 large eggs
- Zest of 1 lemon
- Juice of 1 lemon
- 2 tablespoons poppy seeds
- 1 teaspoon baking soda
- 1/4 teaspoon salt

INSTRUCTIONS:

1. Preheat your oven to 350°F (175°C). Line a muffin tin with paper liners or grease with coconut oil.
2. In a large bowl, whisk together almond flour, coconut flour, baking soda, and salt.
3. In another bowl, whisk together melted coconut oil, honey, eggs, lemon zest, and lemon juice until well combined.
4. Pour the wet ingredients into the dry ingredients and stir until just combined. Do not over mix.
5. Gently fold in poppy seeds until evenly distributed in the batter.
6. Spoon the batter evenly into the prepared muffin tin, filling each cup about 3/4 full.
7. Bake in the preheated oven for 18-20 minutes, or until a toothpick inserted into the center of a muffin comes out clean.
8. Remove from the oven and allow the muffins to cool in the tin for 5 minutes before transferring to a wire rack to cool completely.
9. Once cooled, store in an airtight container at room temperature for up to 3 days, or freeze for longer storage.
10. Enjoy your delightful Almond Flour Lemon Poppy Seed Muffins as a guilt-free treat!

Nutritional Information (per muffin):
Calories: Approximately 180 kcal
Protein: 5g
Fiber: 2g

HEALTH BENEFITS:

Almond flour is a low-carb, high-protein alternative to traditional flour, providing healthy fats and fiber. Lemons add vitamin C and antioxidants, while poppy seeds contribute additional nutrients and fiber. These muffins are a tasty and wholesome option for a balanced dessert.

POINT VALUE:

4

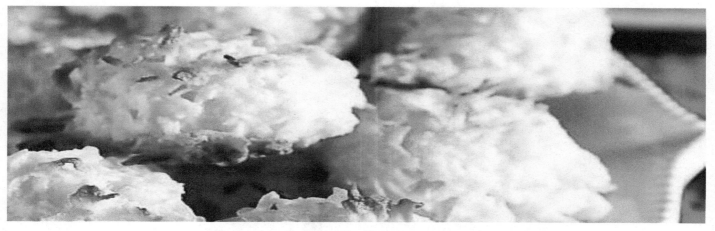

Coconut Macaroons

COOKING TIME: 20 MIN | PREP TIME: 10 MIN | TOTAL TIME: 30 MIN | SERVING SIZE: 12

INGREDIENTS:

- 2 cups unsweetened shredded coconut
- 1/2 cup egg whites (about 4 large eggs)
- 1/4 cup honey
- 1 teaspoon vanilla extract
- 1/4 teaspoon salt

INSTRUCTIONS:

1. Preheat your oven to 325°F (160°C). Line a baking sheet with parchment paper.
2. In a large mixing bowl, combine the shredded coconut, egg whites, honey, vanilla extract, and salt. Mix well until all ingredients are thoroughly combined.
3. Using a tablespoon or small cookie scoop, scoop the coconut mixture and drop it onto the prepared baking sheet, forming small mounds.
4. Bake in the preheated oven for 18-20 minutes, or until the edges of the macaroons are golden brown.
5. Remove from the oven and let the macaroons cool on the baking sheet for 5 minutes.
6. Transfer the macaroons to a wire rack to cool completely.
7. Once cooled, serve and enjoy these delightful Coconut Macaroons!

Nutritional Information (per macaroon):

Calories: Approximately 90 kcal

Protein: 1g

Carbohydrates: 9g

Fiber: 2g

HEALTH BENEFITS:

Coconut is rich in healthy fats, fiber, and minerals like manganese. These macaroons are low in carbohydrates and sugars, making them a light and satisfying dessert that can help curb cravings and support a healthy diet.

POINT VALUE:

3

5

SOUP & SALAD RECIPES

Welcome to the Soup & Salad section of the "Watch Your Weight Cookbook"! Here, you'll find a collection of delicious and nutrient-packed recipes designed to support your weight loss journey. Soups and salads are fantastic options for anyone looking to shed pounds, as they are often low in calories but high in vitamins, minerals, and fiber. These recipes are crafted to keep you feeling full and satisfied without compromising on taste.

In this section, you will discover a variety of recipes, from light and refreshing salads perfect for a quick lunch to hearty soups that can serve as a comforting dinner. Each recipe is carefully curated with a balanced blend of ingredients to ensure you get the most nutritional benefit while enjoying your meal.

Dive into these recipes and enjoy the journey of eating well while watching your weight. Remember, healthy eating is not about restriction but about making choices that nourish your body and soul. Let's get started with some wholesome and delicious soups and salads!

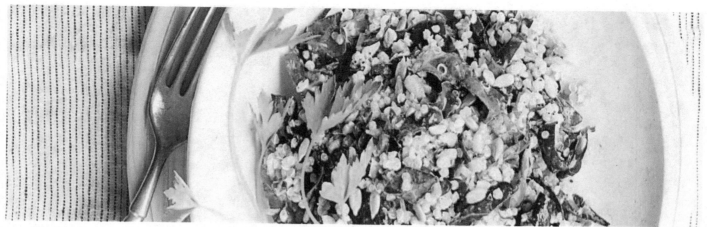

Kale and Quinoa Salad with Lemon Dressing

COOKING TIME: 15 MIN | PREP TIME: 15 MIN | TOTAL TIME: 30 MIN | SERVING SIZE: 4

INGREDIENTS:

- 1 cup quinoa, rinsed
- 2 cups water or vegetable broth
- 4 cups chopped kale leaves, tough stems removed
- 1 cup cherry tomatoes, halved
- 1/2 cup cucumber, diced
- 1/4 cup red onion, thinly sliced
- 1/4 cup fresh parsley, chopped
- 1/4 cup feta cheese, crumbled
- 2 tablespoons olive oil
- 2 tablespoons fresh lemon juice
- 1 teaspoon honey
- Salt and pepper to taste

INSTRUCTIONS:

1. In a medium saucepan, bring 2 cups of water or vegetable broth to a boil. Add quinoa, reduce heat to low, cover, and simmer for 15 minutes, or until quinoa is cooked and water is absorbed. Remove from heat and let it cool.
2. In a large mixing bowl, combine chopped kale leaves, cherry tomatoes, diced cucumber, thinly sliced red onion, and chopped parsley.
3. In a small bowl, whisk together olive oil, fresh lemon juice, honey, salt, and pepper to make the dressing.
4. Add cooked and cooled quinoa to the salad bowl with the vegetables.
5. Pour the lemon dressing over the salad and toss everything together until well combined.
6. Sprinkle crumbled feta cheese over the salad.
7. Serve immediately or refrigerate for 30 minutes to allow flavors to meld before serving.
8. Enjoy your nutritious and flavorful Kale and Quinoa Salad with Lemon Dressing!

Nutritional Information (per serving):

Calories: Approximately 280 kcal
Protein: 9g
Carbohydrates: 34g
Fiber: 5g

HEALTH BENEFITS:

Kale is a nutrient-dense leafy green packed with vitamins A, C, and K, as well as antioxidants and fiber. Quinoa provides complete protein and essential amino acids. The lemon dressing adds vitamin C and enhances flavor, making this salad a nutritious and satisfying option.

POINT VALUE:

4

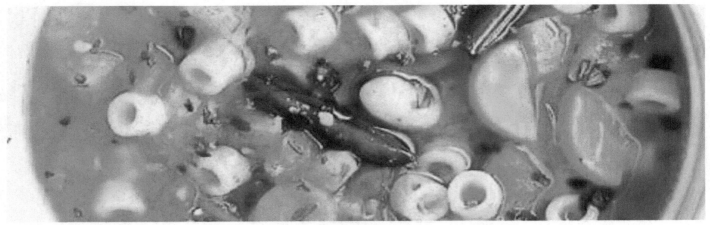

Minestrone Soup with Vegetables and Beans

COOKING TIME: 30 MIN | PREP TIME: 15 MIN | TOTAL TIME: 45 MIN | SERVING SIZE: 6

INGREDIENTS:

- 1 tablespoon olive oil
- 1 medium onion, diced
- 2 cloves garlic, minced
- 2 medium carrots, diced
- 2 celery stalks, diced
- 1 zucchini, diced
- 1 yellow squash, diced
- 1 can (14 oz) diced tomatoes, with juices
- 4 cups low-sodium vegetable broth
- 1 can (15 oz) cannellini beans, drained and rinsed
- 1 teaspoon dried oregano
- 1 teaspoon dried basil
- Salt and pepper to taste
- 2 cups chopped fresh spinach
- 1/2 cup small pasta (such as ditalini or small shells)

HEALTH BENEFITS:

This soup is rich in vegetables, providing a variety of vitamins, minerals, and fiber. Beans add protein and further fiber, promoting satiety and digestive health. Minestrone is low in calories but high in nutrients, making it ideal for weight management.

INSTRUCTIONS:

1. In a large pot or Dutch oven, heat olive oil over medium heat. Add diced onion and cook until translucent, about 3-4 minutes.
2. Add minced garlic and cook for another 1 minute until fragrant.
3. Add diced carrots, celery, zucchini, and yellow squash to the pot. Cook for 5-6 minutes, stirring occasionally, until vegetables begin to soften.
4. Stir in diced tomatoes (with juices) and vegetable broth. Bring to a boil.
5. Reduce heat to low and add cannellini beans, dried oregano, dried basil, salt, and pepper. Simmer uncovered for 15-20 minutes, or until vegetables are tender.
6. In the last 5 minutes of cooking, stir in chopped spinach and small pasta. Cook until pasta is al dente.
7. Taste and adjust seasoning if needed.
8. Serve hot, garnished with freshly grated Parmesan cheese if desired.
9. Enjoy your hearty and nutritious Minestrone Soup with Vegetables and Beans!

Nutritional Information (per serving):

Calories: Approximately 220 kcal

Protein: 9g

Carbohydrates: 38g

Fiber: 8g

POINT VALUE:

4

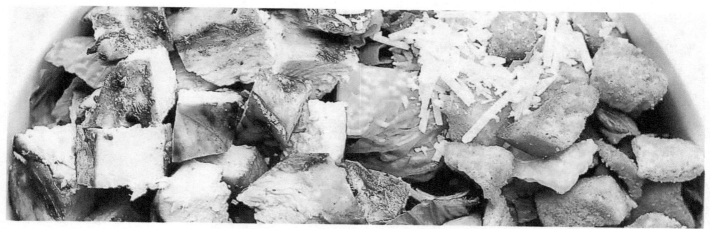

Caesar Salad with Grilled Chicken

COOKING TIME: 15 MIN | PREP TIME: 15 MIN | TOTAL TIME: 30 MIN | SERVING SIZE: 4

INGREDIENTS:

- 2 boneless, skinless chicken breasts
- 1 tablespoon olive oil
- Salt and pepper to taste
- 1 head romaine lettuce, washed and chopped
- 1/2 cup grated Parmesan cheese
- 1/2 cup whole wheat croutons
- Caesar dressing (use a light or reduced-fat version if available)

INSTRUCTIONS:

1. Preheat a grill or grill pan over medium-high heat. Season chicken breasts with olive oil, salt, and pepper.
2. Grill the chicken breasts for about 6-7 minutes per side, or until they reach an internal temperature of 165°F (75°C) and are no longer pink in the center. Remove from heat and let rest for 5 minutes before slicing.
3. While the chicken is resting, prepare the salad. In a large salad bowl, combine chopped romaine lettuce, grated Parmesan cheese, and whole wheat croutons.
4. Slice grilled chicken breasts into thin strips.
5. Add the sliced chicken to the salad bowl.
6. Drizzle Caesar dressing over the salad, starting with a small amount and adding more as desired, tossing gently to coat evenly.
7. Serve immediately and enjoy your nutritious and flavorful Caesar Salad with Grilled Chicken!

Nutritional Information (per serving):

Calories: Approximately 250 kcal

Protein: 28g

Carbohydrates: 10g

Fiber: 3g

HEALTH BENEFITS:

Grilled chicken is a lean source of protein, essential for muscle maintenance and repair. Romaine lettuce is low in calories and high in vitamins A and K. The Caesar dressing and parmesan add flavor while keeping the dish balanced and nutritious.

POINT VALUE:

5

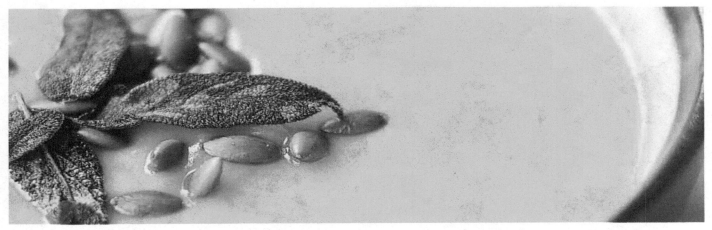

Butternut Squash Soup with Apple and Sage

COOKING TIME: 40 MIN | PREP TIME: 15 MIN | TOTAL TIME: 55 MIN | SERVING SIZE: 6

INGREDIENTS:

- 1 medium butternut squash, peeled, seeded, and cubed (about 4 cups)
- 2 apples, peeled, cored, and chopped
- 1 onion, chopped
- 4 cups low-sodium vegetable broth
- 1 cup unsweetened almond milk (or low-fat milk)
- 2 tablespoons olive oil
- 2 cloves garlic, minced
- 1 tablespoon fresh sage leaves, chopped (plus extra for garnish)
- Salt and pepper to taste

INSTRUCTIONS:

1. In a large pot or Dutch oven, heat olive oil over medium heat. Add chopped onion and cook for 3-4 minutes until softened.
2. Add minced garlic and chopped sage leaves to the pot. Cook for another 1-2 minutes until fragrant.
3. Add cubed butternut squash and chopped apples to the pot. Stir to combine with the onion mixture.
4. Pour in the vegetable broth and bring to a boil. Reduce heat to low, cover, and simmer for 20-25 minutes, or until the butternut squash and apples are tender.
5. Remove the pot from heat and let it cool slightly.
6. Using an immersion blender, blend the soup until smooth and creamy. Alternatively, transfer the soup in batches to a blender and blend until smooth, then return to the pot.
7. Stir in almond milk (or low-fat milk) until well combined. Season with salt and pepper to taste.
8. Return the pot to the stove and heat gently over low heat until warmed through.
9. Ladle the Butternut Squash Soup into serving bowls. Garnish with additional chopped sage leaves if desired.
10. Serve hot and enjoy this comforting and nutritious Butternut Squash Soup with Apple and Sage!

Nutritional Information (per serving): Calories: Approximately 180 kcal, Protein: 3g, Carbohydrates: 30g, Fiber: 6g

HEALTH BENEFITS:

Butternut squash is high in vitamins A and C, fiber, and antioxidants. Apples add natural sweetness and additional fiber, while sage provides anti-inflammatory properties. This soup is comforting and nutrient-rich, supporting overall health and weight loss.

POINT VALUE:

4

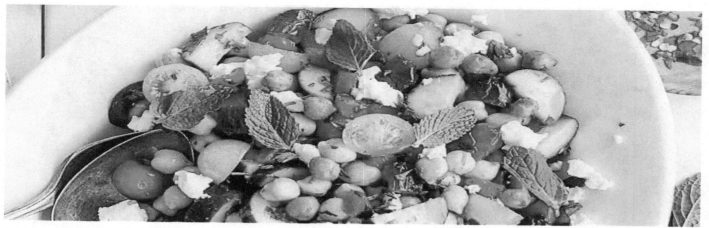

Mediterranean Chickpea Salad with Feta

COOKING TIME: 0 MIN | PREP TIME: 15 MIN | TOTAL TIME: 15 MIN | SERVING SIZE: 4

INGREDIENTS:

- 1 can (15 oz) chickpeas, drained and rinsed
- 1 cucumber, diced
- 1 cup cherry tomatoes, halved
- 1/2 red onion, thinly sliced
- 1/4 cup Kalamata olives, pitted and sliced
- 2 oz feta cheese, crumbled
- 1/4 cup fresh parsley, chopped
- 2 tablespoons extra virgin olive oil
- 2 tablespoons red wine vinegar
- 1 teaspoon dried oregano
- Salt and pepper to taste

INSTRUCTIONS:

1. In a large salad bowl, combine the chickpeas, diced cucumber, cherry tomatoes, red onion, and Kalamata olives, crumbled feta cheese, and chopped parsley.
2. In a small bowl, whisk together the extra virgin olive oil, red wine vinegar, dried oregano, salt, and pepper.
3. Pour the dressing over the salad ingredients in the bowl.
4. Toss gently to combine all ingredients and coat them evenly with the dressing.
5. Taste and adjust seasoning with salt and pepper if needed.
6. Serve immediately or refrigerate for 30 minutes to allow flavors to meld before serving.
7. Enjoy your refreshing and nutritious Mediterranean Chickpea Salad with Feta!

Nutritional Information (per serving):

Calories: Approximately 250 kcal

Protein: 9g

Carbohydrates: 24g

Fiber: 7g

HEALTH BENEFITS:

Chickpeas are a great source of plant-based protein and fiber, aiding in digestion and satiety. Feta cheese adds calcium and a savory flavor, while the Mediterranean vegetables provide a variety of vitamins and minerals. This salad is filling and nutritious.

POINT VALUE:

4

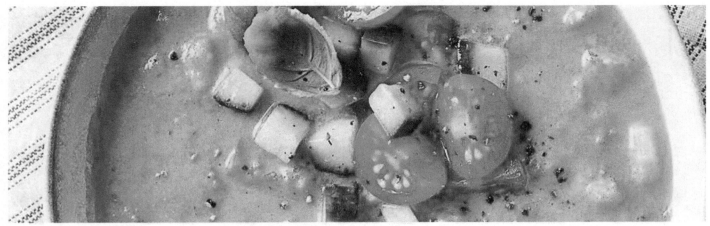

Gazpacho with Cucumber and Tomato

COOKING TIME: 0 MIN | PREP TIME: 15 MIN | TOTAL TIME: 15 MIN | SERVING SIZE: 4

INGREDIENTS:

- 4 large tomatoes, chopped
- 1 cucumber, peeled, seeded, and chopped
- 1 red bell pepper, seeded and chopped
- 1/2 red onion, chopped
- 2 cloves garlic, minced
- 1/4 cup fresh parsley leaves
- 2 tablespoons red wine vinegar
- 2 tablespoons olive oil
- 1/2 teaspoon salt
- 1/4 teaspoon black pepper
- 1/4 teaspoon cayenne pepper (optional, adjust to taste)

INSTRUCTIONS:

1. In a blender or food processor, combine the chopped tomatoes, cucumber, red bell pepper, red onion, garlic, and parsley leaves.
2. Blend on high until smooth and well combined.
3. Add red wine vinegar, olive oil, salt, black pepper, and cayenne pepper (if using). Blend again until all ingredients are thoroughly mixed.
4. Taste and adjust seasoning if needed.
5. Transfer the gazpacho to a large bowl or container and refrigerate for at least 1 hour to chill.
6. Serve the chilled Gazpacho with Cucumber and Tomato in individual bowls or glasses.
7. Optionally, garnish with additional chopped cucumber, tomato, or parsley leaves.
8. Enjoy your refreshing and nutritious Gazpacho as a light and satisfying soup!

Nutritional Information (per serving):

Calories: Approximately 100 kcal

Protein: 2g

Carbohydrates: 10g

Fiber: 3g

HEALTH BENEFITS:

Gazpacho is a cold soup made with tomatoes, cucumbers, bell peppers, and onions, all of which are low in calories and high in vitamins, antioxidants, and fiber. This refreshing soup is hydrating and supports digestive health and weight loss.

POINT VALUE:

2

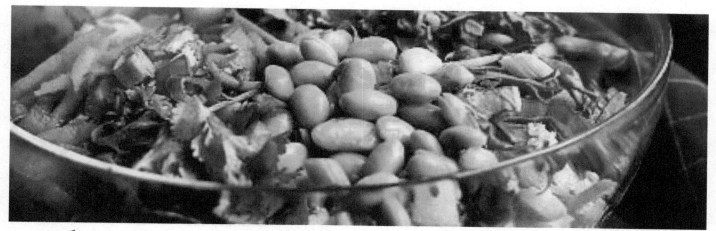

Thai Quinoa Salad with Peanut Dressing

COOKING TIME: 20 MIN | PREP TIME: 15 MIN | TOTAL TIME: 35 MIN | SERVING SIZE: 4

INGREDIENTS:

- 1 cup quinoa, rinsed
- 2 cups water
- 1 red bell pepper, diced
- 1 cup shredded carrots
- 1/2 cup edamame, shelled
- 1/4 cup chopped fresh cilantro
- 1/4 cup chopped green onions
- 1/4 cup peanuts, chopped (optional garnish)

For the Peanut Dressing:
- 1/4 cup natural peanut butter
- 2 tablespoons soy sauce (low-sodium)
- 2 tablespoons rice vinegar
- 1 tablespoon honey
- 1 tablespoon fresh lime juice
- 1 teaspoon sesame oil
- 1 teaspoon grated fresh ginger
- 1 clove garlic, minced
- Water (as needed to thin dressing)

HEALTH BENEFITS:

Quinoa is a complete protein, and the vegetables in the salad provide a range of vitamins, minerals, and fiber. The peanut dressing adds healthy fats and protein, making this salad flavorful and balanced, perfect for sustaining energy and promoting weight loss.

INSTRUCTIONS:

1. In a medium saucepan, bring 2 cups of water to a boil. Add the quinoa, reduce heat to low, cover, and simmer for 15 minutes or until the quinoa is cooked and water is absorbed. Remove from heat and let it sit covered for 5 minutes. Fluff with a fork and let it cool.
2. In a large bowl, combine the cooked quinoa, diced red bell pepper, shredded carrots, edamame, chopped cilantro, and green onions.
3. In a small bowl, whisk together the peanut butter, soy sauce, rice vinegar, honey, lime juice, sesame oil, grated ginger, and minced garlic until smooth. Add water, 1 tablespoon at a time, to thin the dressing to your desired consistency.
4. Pour the peanut dressing over the quinoa and vegetables. Toss gently to coat everything evenly with the dressing.
5. Garnish with chopped peanuts if desired.
6. Serve chilled or at room temperature, and enjoy this flavorful Thai Quinoa Salad with Peanut Dressing!

Nutritional Information (per serving):
Calories: Approximately 350 kcal
Protein: 12g
Carbohydrates: 44g
Fiber: 7g

POINT VALUE:

5

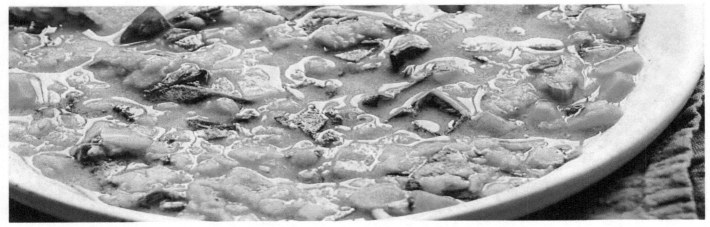

Spinach and Lentil Soup

COOKING TIME: 30 MIN | PREP TIME: 10 MIN | TOTAL TIME: 40 MIN | SERVING SIZE: 6

INGREDIENTS:

- 1 cup dried green lentils, rinsed
- 1 onion, diced
- 2 carrots, diced
- 2 celery stalks, diced
- 3 cloves garlic, minced
- 1 teaspoon ground cumin
- 1/2 teaspoon ground turmeric
- 1/2 teaspoon ground paprika
- 6 cups vegetable broth (low sodium)
- 4 cups fresh spinach leaves
- 2 tablespoons olive oil
- Salt and pepper to taste

INSTRUCTIONS:

1. In a large pot or Dutch oven, heat olive oil over medium heat. Add diced onion, carrots, and celery. Cook for 5-6 minutes until vegetables are softened.
2. Add minced garlic, ground cumin, ground turmeric, and ground paprika to the pot. Stir well and cook for 1-2 minutes until fragrant.
3. Add rinsed green lentils to the pot and stir to combine with the vegetables and spices.
4. Pour in vegetable broth and bring to a boil. Reduce heat to low, cover, and simmer for 20-25 minutes, or until lentils are tender.
5. Stir in fresh spinach leaves and cook for an additional 2-3 minutes until spinach is wilted.
6. Season with salt and pepper to taste.
7. Remove from heat and let the soup cool slightly before serving.
8. Ladle the Spinach and Lentil Soup into bowls and serve hot.
9. Enjoy your hearty and nutritious Spinach and Lentil Soup!

Nutritional Information (per serving):
Calories: Approximately 200 kcal

Protein: 10g

Carbohydrates: 30g

Fiber: 12g

HEALTH BENEFITS:
Spinach is rich in iron, vitamins A and C, and antioxidants. Lentils are high in protein, fiber, and essential nutrients like folate and iron. This soup is nutrient-dense, low in calories, and supports digestive health and weight management.

POINT VALUE:

4

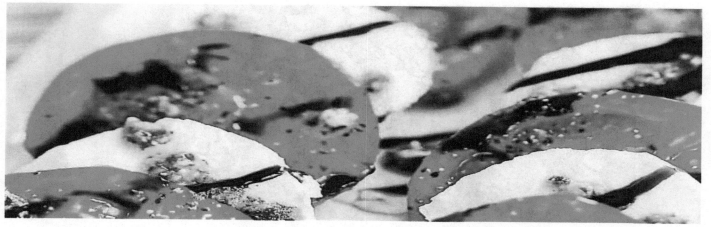

Caprese Salad with Pesto Dressing

PREP TIME: 15 MIN | TOTAL TIME: 15 MIN | SERVING SIZE: 2

INGREDIENTS:

- 2 medium tomatoes, sliced
- 1 ball fresh mozzarella cheese, sliced
- 1 cup fresh basil leaves
- 2 tablespoons prepared pesto sauce
- 1 tablespoon balsamic vinegar
- 1 tablespoon olive oil
- Salt and pepper to taste

INSTRUCTIONS:

1. Arrange the sliced tomatoes and mozzarella cheese alternately on a serving platter.
2. Scatter fresh basil leaves over the tomatoes and mozzarella.
3. In a small bowl, whisk together pesto sauce, balsamic vinegar, and olive oil until well combined.
4. Drizzle the pesto dressing over the Caprese salad.
5. Season with salt and pepper to taste.
6. Serve immediately and enjoy your refreshing and flavorful Caprese Salad with Pesto Dressing!

Nutritional Information (per serving):
Calories: Approximately 250 kcal
Protein: 12g
Carbohydrates: 8g
Fiber: 2g

HEALTH BENEFITS:

Tomatoes provide vitamins C and K and antioxidants, while mozzarella adds protein and calcium. The pesto dressing, made from basil and pine nuts, offers healthy fats and additional vitamins. This salad is light, refreshing, and nutritious.

POINT VALUE:

4

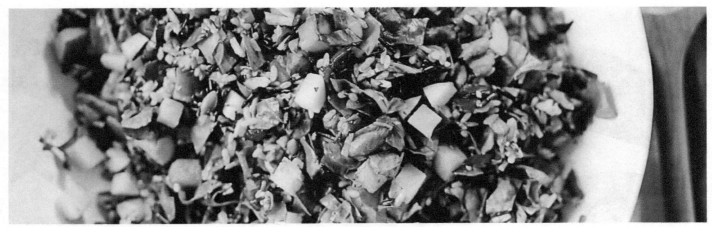

Sweet Potato and Kale Salad with Maple Vinaigrette

COOKING TIME: 25 MIN | PREP TIME: 15 MIN | TOTAL TIME: 40 MIN | SERVING SIZE: 4

INGREDIENTS:

- 2 medium sweet potatoes, peeled and diced
- 6 cups kale leaves, chopped
- 1/4 cup dried cranberries
- 1/4 cup chopped pecans
- 1/4 cup crumbled feta cheese (optional, not included in point value)
- 2 tablespoons olive oil
- 1 tablespoon apple cider vinegar
- 1 tablespoon pure maple syrup
- Salt and pepper to taste

INSTRUCTIONS:

1. Preheat your oven to 400°F (200°C). Line a baking sheet with parchment paper.
2. Toss diced sweet potatoes with 1 tablespoon of olive oil, salt, and pepper. Spread evenly on the prepared baking sheet.
3. Roast the sweet potatoes in the preheated oven for 20-25 minutes, or until tender and lightly browned. Remove from oven and let cool slightly.
4. In a large salad bowl, combine chopped kale, roasted sweet potatoes, dried cranberries, and chopped pecans.
5. In a small bowl, whisk together remaining 1 tablespoon of olive oil, apple cider vinegar, and maple syrup to make the vinaigrette.
6. Pour the maple vinaigrette over the salad and toss gently to coat all ingredients.
7. Divide the salad into serving bowls.
8. If using, sprinkle crumbled feta cheese over the top of each serving.
9. Serve immediately and enjoy your nutritious and flavorful Sweet Potato and Kale Salad!

Nutritional Information (per serving):

Calories: Approximately 250 kcal

Protein: 4g

Carbohydrates: 36g

Fiber: 5g

HEALTH BENEFITS:

Sweet potatoes are high in vitamins A and C, fiber, and antioxidants. Kale is a super food rich in vitamins, minerals, and fiber. The maple vinaigrette adds a touch of natural sweetness without excessive calories. This salad is hearty, nutritious, and supports weight management.

POINT VALUE:

4

14 DAYS MEAL PLAN

Day 1
- **Breakfast**: Greek Yogurt Parfait with Fresh Berries
- **Lunch**: Grilled Chicken Salad with Balsamic Vinaigrette
- **Dinner**: Baked Salmon with Dill and Lemon

Day 2
- **Breakfast**: Spinach and Mushroom Egg White Omelette
- **Lunch**: Quinoa Stuffed Bell Peppers
- **Dinner**: Spaghetti Squash with Turkey Bolognese

Day 3
- **Breakfast**: Whole Grain Pancakes with Banana and Walnuts
- **Lunch**: Lentil and Vegetable Soup
- **Dinner**: Grilled Lemon Herb Chicken with Quinoa

Day 4
- **Breakfast**: Avocado Toast with Poached Egg
- **Lunch**: Asian-Inspired Tofu Stir-Fry
- **Dinner**: Stuffed Portobello Mushrooms with Spinach and Feta

Day 5
- **Breakfast**: Quinoa Breakfast Bowl with Almond Butter and Fruit
- **Lunch**: Chickpea Salad with Lemon Tahini Dressing
- **Dinner**: Lemon Garlic Shrimp with Zucchini Noodles

Day 6
- **Breakfast**: Chia Seed Pudding with Berries
- **Lunch**: Caprese Salad with Balsamic Glaze
- **Dinner**: Turkey and Sweet Potato Skillet

Day 7
- **Breakfast**: Green Smoothie with Spinach and Pineapple
- **Lunch**: Turkey and Spinach Meatballs in Marinara Sauce
- **Dinner**: Eggplant Parmesan with Whole Wheat Pasta

Day 8
- **Breakfast**: Veggie Egg White Scramble
- **Lunch**: Mediterranean Veggie Wrap with Hummus
- **Dinner**: Coconut Curry Chicken with Cauliflower Rice

Day 9
- **Breakfast**: Oatmeal with Apples and Cinnamon
- **Lunch**: Cauliflower Fried Rice with Shrimp
- **Dinner**: Quinoa and Black Bean Stuffed Peppers

Day 10
- Breakfast: Cottage Cheese and Fruit Bowl
- Lunch: Caesar Salad with Grilled Chicken
- Dinner: Baked Chicken Breast with Rosemary and Garlic

Day 11
- **Breakfast**: Baked Apple with Cinnamon and Walnuts
- **Lunch**: Butternut Squash Soup with Apple and Sage
- **Dinner**: Zucchini Noodles with Pesto and Cherry Tomatoes

Day 12
- **Breakfast**: Banana Oatmeal Cookies
- **Lunch**: Mediterranean Chickpea Salad with Feta
- **Dinner**: Lentil and Sweet Potato Shepherd's Pie

Day 13
- **Breakfast**: Mixed Berry Frozen Yogurt
- **Lunch**: Thai Quinoa Salad with Peanut Dressing
- **Dinner**: Grilled Veggie Skewers with Quinoa

Day 14
- **Breakfast**: Dark Chocolate Avocado Mousse
- **Lunch**: Spinach and Lentil Soup
- **Dinner**: Cauliflower Crust Pizza with Veggies

Frequently Asked Questions (FAQs)

How do the point values work in this cookbook?
The point values assigned to each recipe in this cookbook are designed to help you track your daily food intake while supporting your weight loss journey. These values are based on a balanced approach to nutrition, focusing on portion control and healthy ingredient choices.

Can I customize recipes to fit my dietary preferences or restrictions?
Absolutely! Many recipes in this cookbook are versatile and can be adapted to accommodate various dietary needs, such as vegetarian, gluten-free, or dairy-free. Feel free to make substitutions or adjustments to suit your preferences while keeping the overall nutritional balance in mind.

How can this cookbook help me achieve my weight loss goals?
This cookbook provides a collection of delicious and nutritious recipes that are lower in calories and points, making it easier to manage your daily food intake while enjoying satisfying meals. By following the recipes and portion guidelines, you can adopt healthier eating habits that support sustainable weight loss.

Are the recipes in this cookbook family-friendly?
Yes, many of the recipes in this cookbook are designed to appeal to a wide range of tastes and preferences, making them suitable for the whole family. You can adjust serving sizes or pair dishes with complementary sides to accommodate everyone at the table.

How do I navigate the points system if I'm new to tracking food intake?
The cookbook includes an introduction that explains how the points system works and provides guidance on calculating and tracking points. Over time, you'll become more familiar with the point values of different foods and how they fit into your daily or weekly goals.

Are the ingredients used in the recipes easy to find in regular grocery stores?
Yes, the recipes feature commonly available ingredients that can be found in most grocery stores. The focus is on using fresh, whole foods to maximize nutritional value and flavor without requiring hard-to-find or specialty items.

Can I use this cookbook if I'm not following a specific weight loss program?
Absolutely! While the recipes in this cookbook are designed with weight loss goals in mind and use a points system for guidance, they can be enjoyed by anyone looking to maintain a balanced and nutritious diet. The emphasis is on wholesome ingredients and delicious flavors that promote overall health.

How can I stay motivated to cook and eat healthy meals from this cookbook?
To stay motivated, try meal planning and involving family or friends in cooking and enjoying meals together. Celebrate your progress and achievements along the way, and remember that small, consistent changes lead to long-term success in achieving your health and weight goals.

Are there tips in the cookbook for portion control and mindful eating?
Yes, the cookbook includes tips and suggestions for portion control, mindful eating practices, and strategies to manage cravings. These resources can help you develop healthier eating habits and make informed choices about food intake.

Is there nutritional information provided for each recipe?
Yes, each recipe in the cookbook includes detailed nutritional information per serving, including calories, protein, carbohydrates, fiber, sugars, fat, saturated fat, cholesterol, sodium, and potassium. This information helps you make informed decisions about your food choices.

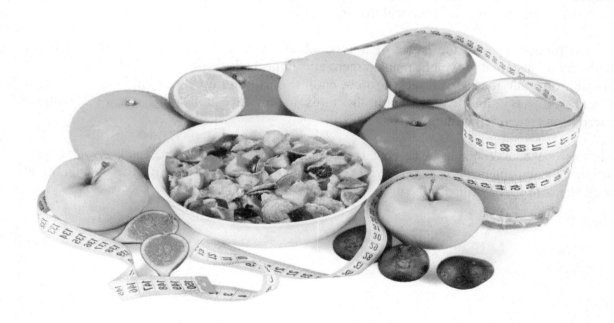

Conclusion

In concluding our culinary journey through the "Watch Your Weight Cookbook," we've embarked on a path to not just healthier eating but a lifestyle transformation. From the very first page, where we introduced the concept of mindful eating and the point-based system designed to guide us, to exploring a plethora of nutritious recipes across breakfasts, lunches, dinners, and delightful desserts, this cookbook has been a companion on our quest for wellness.

Each recipe meticulously crafted not only for flavor but also with your weight loss goals in mind, incorporating ingredients that nourish and satisfy. Whether it was savoring the refreshing Veggie Egg White Scramble at breakfast or relishing the aromatic Coconut Curry Chicken with Cauliflower Rice for dinner, every dish offered a balance of taste and nutrition.

We delved into the art of healthy cooking, understanding the importance of portion control, mindful choices, and the benefits of incorporating whole foods into our diet. The FAQs addressed common queries, guiding us through the nuances of the points system, customization options, and practical tips for success.

As we flipped through the pages of this cookbook, we discovered not just recipes but a pathway to sustainable weight management and improved well-being. Whether you're just starting on your journey or seeking new culinary inspirations, the "Watch Your Weight Cookbook" has equipped you with the tools to embrace a healthier lifestyle without sacrificing taste or enjoyment.

Let this cookbook continue to be your trusted companion in the kitchen, guiding you towards achieving and maintaining your weight loss goals with delicious meals that nourish both body and soul. Here's to a future filled with vibrant health and culinary delights!

67335556R00044